DO YOU KNOW . . . .

- Dietary fat and high cholesterol play an important role in causing prostate problems.

- Three quicker, safer medical procedures are under development to replace traditional surgical approaches to prostate problems.

- Clinical trials have established the value of essential fatty acids in the treatment of prostate disease . . . and two supplements can supply all you need.

- Homeopathic medicines were found effective for up to 95% of prostate patients experiencing groin and perineal pain.

- Hyperthermia, or the use of heat to kill cancer cells, can be combined with radiation to shrink tumors faster . . . and with less radiation.

- Stress can cause a release of hormones in the body that are injurious to prostate tissues . . . and progressive relaxation may be the best antidote.

FIND OUT MORE IN . . . .
**NATURAL MEDICINE FOR PROSTATE
PROBLEMS**

Books available from the Dell Natural Medicine Library:

NATURAL MEDICINE FOR HEART DISEASE

NATURAL MEDICINE FOR BREAST CANCER

NATURAL MEDICINE FOR ARTHRITIS

NATURAL MEDICINE FOR DIABETES

NATURAL MEDICINE FOR BACK PAIN

NATURAL MEDICINE FOR PROSTATE PROBLEMS

NATURAL MEDICINE FOR WEIGHT LOSS

NATURAL MEDICINE FOR COLDS AND FLU

NATURAL MEDICINE FOR PMS

NATURAL MEDICINE FOR SUPER IMMUNITY

THE DELL
NATURAL MEDICINE LIBRARY

NATURAL MEDICINE FOR
PROSTATE PROBLEMS

Ron Falcone

Foreword by Roy B. Kupsinel, M.D.

A Lynn Sonberg Book

A Dell Book

Published by
Dell Publishing
a division of
Bantam Doubleday Dell Publishing Group, Inc.
1540 Broadway
New York, New York 10036

IMPORTANT NOTE: Neither this nor any other book should be used as a substitute for professional medical care or treatment. It is advisable to seek the guidance of a physician or other qualified health practitioner before implementing any of the approaches to health suggested in this book. This book was written to provide selected information to the public concerning conventional and alternative medical treatments for prostate problems. Research in this field is ongoing and subject to interpretation. Although we have made all reasonable efforts to include the most up-to-date and accurate information in this book, there is no guarantee that what we know about this complex subject won't change with time. The reader should bear in mind that this book is not intended to take the place of medical advice from a trained medical professional. Readers are advised to consult a physician or other qualified health professional regarding treatment of all of their health problems. Neither the publisher, the producer, nor the author takes any responsibility for any possible consequences from any treatment, action, or application of medicine or preparation by any person reading or following the information in this book. The names and identifying characteristics of the patients mentioned in this book have been changed to protect their privacy.

ISBN: 0-440-22524-8

Published by arrangement with
Lynn Sonberg Book Associates
10 West 86th Street
New York, NY 10024

Printed in the United States of America
Published simultaneously in Canada
June 1998

10 9 8 7 6 5 4 3 2 1

OPM

CONTENTS

Foreword by Roy B. Kupsinel, M.D.   vii

Introduction   xi

Chapter One: What You Need to Know About Traditional Treatments   1

Chapter Two: Vitamins, Minerals, and Other Supplements   11

Chapter Three: Herb and Plant Remedies   26

Chapter Four: Self-treatment with Homeopathy   46

Chapter Five: Helping Your Prostate Through Diet   55

Chapter Six: Special Exercises, Massage, and Hydrotherapy   76

Chapter Seven: Sex and Your Prostate   89

Chapter Eight: What You Need to Know About Prostate Cancer   95

Chapter Nine: Complementary Approaches for Treating Prostate Cancer   107

Chapter Ten: Putting a Complementary Program into Practice   133

Appendix 1 (Recommended Nutrient Guidelines)   149

Appendix 2 (Important Resources)   153

References   162

Glossary   170

Index   179

FOREWORD

The timing of Ron Falcone's excellent book, *Natural Medicine for Prostate Problems,* couldn't be better. On the one hand, awareness of prostate disease, which afflicts millions of men over the age of fifty, has grown rapidly over the last few years. At the same time, more and more consumers— and medical professionals—are turning to natural medicines as an adjunct to conventional medical care.

This book is a comprehensive, well-researched, and easy-to-understand primer on prostate disease, both benign and cancerous. After introducing the reader to the most commonly used methods of diagnosis and traditional treatments, the author moves on to the main focus of the book: natural medicines. For example, the role of vitamins, minerals, herbs, and other substances that affect prostate function are explored in clear detail; how and when to take these substances are also clearly explained.

The author presents a comprehensive chapter on homeopathy and explains precisely which homeopathic medicines should be taken and in what dosages.

Since the role of diet and prostate health is so important and has gotten much scientific attention in recent years, Mr. Falcone's chapter on this subject will be found especially beneficial; sample diets, foods to avoid, and foods to choose are all examined. In addition, there are diet guidelines that can be used in the treatment of specific prostate conditions.

The book also discusses "time-honored" healing strategies such as special exercises, reflexology, and water therapies that have been used for years to treat various prostate conditions. And the connection between sex and prostate health—an intriguing subject that's not been given sufficient treatment in most books—is examined.

Of course, no book on the prostate would be complete without an examination of one of the most important health issues facing men today: prostate cancer. In fact, 200,000 American men will be diagnosed with this disease every year, and a majority will show some evidence of cancer later in life.

Mr. Falcone provides a thorough explanation of what prostate cancer is, how it's diagnosed, and what present-day medical strategies are being used to treat the disease. In addition, he offers a sensible and balanced look at the many natural medicines that can be used alongside traditional cancer therapies, including therapeutic diets, high-dose vitamins, adjuvant vaccine programs, herbal therapies, and other strategies that are being used with varying degrees of success by complementary health practitioners.

Important as natural medicines are in the treatment of prostate disease, the ultimate goal is to prevent problems from starting in the first place. Fortunately, such problems can often be avoided by paying careful attention to diet, lifestyle, and nutrient balance.

In *Natural Medicine for Prostate Problems,* you'll find a number of key guidelines on the all-important issue of prevention. I highly recommend *Natural Medicine for Prostate Problems.* Easy to use and reassuring to the lay reader, it will also help raise the awareness and understanding of professionals who are interested in learning more about the many ways that natural medicine can treat prostate problems—or prevent them from developing in the first place.

Roy B. Kupsinel, M.D.
Medical Director, Lost Horizon Health Awareness Center
Oviedo, Florida

INTRODUCTION

Each year in the United States, 200,000 men are diagnosed with prostate cancer, and nearly 40,000 succumb to the disease. But for every cancer that's diagnosed, there are five times more cases of benign prostate enlargement and inflammation. In fact, these disorders are *so common* that they are almost considered an inevitable part of life.

If you've been diagnosed with prostate disease, you can benefit from the natural medicines described in this book. These medicines are generally safe and nontoxic, and they include vitamins and minerals, herbs and plant substances, homeopathic remedies, special diets, and exercise and massage therapies.

Exactly what can natural medicines do for you? Here are just a few examples: Special vitamins and minerals can help lower harmful levels of testosterone and other hormones that harm your prostate; medicinal herbs and plants can reduce swelling and inflammation; homeopathic medicines can alleviate prostate-related symptoms safely and without side effects; and special diets can bolster your body's healing forces and speed up your recovery from prostate disease.

Natural medicines can also offer you much benefit if you've been diagnosed with prostate cancer. Specific nutrients, herbs, diet therapies, and other natural strategies can optimize your cancer-fighting ability and safeguard you against the damaging effects of toxic cancer treatments. In addition, complementary cancer therapies are now available that work with, not against, the body's healing forces (we'll provide you with updated information on complementary therapies later in the book).

The use of natural medicines for prostate problems and for other diseases is no longer being viewed as health "faddism." In fact, an ever-increasing number of Americans are now taking it upon themselves to seek and investigate natural treatments long considered at odds with orthodox medicine. In a recent Gallup poll, for example, one third of adults questioned revealed that they had sought natural treatment for a wide range of diseases. The adults were between the ages of twenty-five and forty-nine, and most had higher levels of education and income.

Surprisingly, physicians who practice traditional medicine are also getting involved—as seen by their increasing enrollment in health organizations that offer natural therapies. Such a change in thinking by the medical community wasn't even thought possible a few decades ago.

In a move seen by many as a further boon to the natural health movement, the National Institutes of Health (NIH) recently established the Office of Alternative Medicine (OAM). The OAM investigates the positive claims being made for remedies discussed in this book and elsewhere, and in many cases, evidence supporting the use of such treatments for prostate cancer is being established.

Always remember that natural medicines, helpful as they are, are not meant to be used in place of the established medical treatments. You should always consult a physician before undertaking any natural program—especially if you are experiencing any symptoms of prostate disease.

How to Use This Book

Whether you have prostate disease or are simply concerned about preventing it, the information in this book will help you meet your objectives safely and effectively.

Before delving into natural healing strategies for the prostate, we'll examine what the prostate is, how it works, and what can go wrong with it; we'll also talk about the traditional treatments that are used for prostate disease. See **Chapter 1** for full details.

Recent studies have shown that certain vitamins and minerals help the prostate by lowering harmful levels of testosterone in its tissues—while also improving the body's healing capabilities. In addition, protective nutrients are known to help the body reduce or even eliminate harmful toxins and pollutants that can injure the prostate. Essential fatty acids and amino acids are also showing positive effects on prostate function. In **Chapter 2,** everything you'll need to know about prostate-healing vitamins, minerals, and other nutrients will be examined. (A more detailed supplement program is included in **Appendix 1.**)

In recent years, the native Florida plant saw palmetto has received lots of attention for its favorable role in treating benign prostatic hyperplasia, or BPH. In addition, there are a number of other useful herb and plant substances that can be used in combination with saw palmetto. These plant combinations often increase the odds of a cure for BPH and may help with infectious conditions as well. A full discussion of herbal remedies—including those used in Western medicine and in traditional Chinese medicine—is provided in **Chapter 3.**

Plant substances are also used in the manufacture of *homeopathic medicines,* and these too are being used with claims of success for many different prostate disorders. See

Chapter 4 for complete information on homeopathy and the prostate.

The role of proper diet and its effect on prostate health is gaining importance among researchers. One key factor believed to directly affect the prostate is dietary fat and the free-radical damage that's associated with it. (Cancer and lowered immunity are also both linked to fat intake.) Processed and starchy foods, food additives, a lack of dietary fiber, and other factors are also thought to play important roles in prostate disease. See **Chapter 5** for a full discussion.

Time-honored methods for healing the prostate—including special exercises, massage therapies, and hot or cold sitz baths—will be examined in **Chapter 6.**

The influence of sexual activity on prostate health has long been a subject of interest. Some physicians believe that more frequent sex is better for the prostate, while others recommend sexual "rest periods" to allow the prostate a chance to heal; this issue and others will be examined in **Chapter 7.**

Perhaps one of the greatest areas of concern today is prostate cancer. Newer treatment strategies are being developed to conquer this much-feared disease; there are also a number of natural medicines that can serve as useful complements to the standard treatments. Everything you'll need to know about prostate cancer and current treatments will be discussed in **Chapter 8.**

Natural medicines for prostate cancer—including therapeutic diets, high-dose vitamins, adjuvant vaccine programs, and herbal therapies—will be examined in **Chapter 9.**

In **Chapter 10,** we'll provide real-life examples of how three men with prostate disease went about devising their own complementary treatment program; we'll also include valuable information on how to find a complementary health practitioner.

And in the book's two **appendixes,** you'll find complete nutrient guidelines for the prostate and additional resource information.

Starting Your Own Program

When should you begin a complementary program for your prostate? And what type of program should you pursue? There are actually several answers to these questions—depending on your present state of health.

If you are in good health and haven't been diagnosed with a prostate problem, you'll want to give consideration to a *preventive program.* As described earlier, prostate disease is all too common, and the prostate seldom becomes noticed until problems start. By following the general guidelines for prostate health outlined in this book, you can go a long way toward preventing unnecessary suffering and discomfort later on.

If you *are* experiencing symptoms of prostate enlargement or inflammation, you'll need to see your doctor before undertaking a complementary program. Then if the doctor finds a diagnosis of prostate disease, he may want to prescribe a course of treatment or simply observe you to see if symptoms worsen or improve (this is known as watchful waiting). But whether you ultimately receive medical treatment or not, the natural medicines recommended in this book can help increase your chances of a fuller and speedier recovery.

Before You Begin

It is always wise to consult with your supervising physician before starting a complementary treatment program. After all, some treatments may not be completely harmless (even though they are completely *natural*), so it is always a good idea to discuss their use beforehand.

If your physician isn't comfortable with the idea of complementary treatments or doesn't seem willing to engage in a serious discussion about them, consider seeking out a second or third opinion from a nutritionally oriented physician or naturopathic doctor.

One more point bears mention. Admittedly, there's lots of information contained in this book, and it may, at times, seem a bit overwhelming. But by carefully reading through the recommendations that best apply to your medical situation, and by working closely with a qualified health practitioner, you'll be able to easily plan a treatment program that suits your individual needs.

CHAPTER ONE

What You Need to Know About Traditional Treatments

While prostate cancer has rightfully become one of the most publicized health issues of the 1990s, men are *five times* more likely to develop *benign* prostate diseases such as enlargement and inflammation. In fact, *1,000,000* American men are diagnosed with these conditions annually.

Benign prostate disease is so common that it is often considered an inevitable part of life. But fortunately, a variety of natural medicines and healing strategies—including vitamins, minerals, herbs and plant substances, homeopathic remedies, diets, exercise, and therapeutic massage—can help alleviate or even reverse prostate disease. These same medicines can also be used to *prevent* diseases from ever starting in the first place.

Before we explain natural treatments, it's important to understand what the prostate is, what can go wrong with it, and how the medical profession is currently treating prostate diseases.

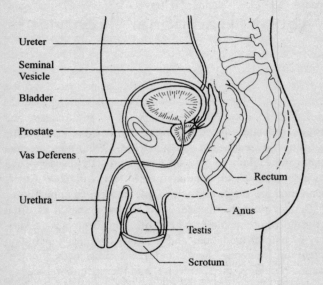

Ureter

Seminal
Vesicle

Bladder

Prostate

Vas Deferens

Urethra

Rectum

Anus

Testis

Scrotum

Understanding Your Prostate

Although it weighs only about one ounce, your prostate plays an important role in many key functions, including healthy urination and sexual performance.

The prostate is a walnut-shaped gland that's located directly beneath the bladder (see illustration). When urine passes from the bladder, it travels into a tube that goes through the middle of the prostate (called the *prostatic urethra*). If the prostate is enlarged, the urethra can become closed off, making urination difficult or in some cases almost impossible (more on this later in the chapter).

There is another tube that enters the prostate, and it's called the *vas deferens*. Originating in the testicles, the vas deferens goes up and around the top of the bladder, and then down into the prostate, where it too joins the prostatic urethra. When sperm is ejaculated, it travels through the vas deferens, the prostatic urethra, and then out through the penis.

The prostate plays two key roles in the release of healthy sperm. First, sperm is nourished in the prostate by a special protein-rich liquid known as *seminal fluid;* second, sperm is given its push out of the body by contractions occurring within the prostate.

The prostate also has a crucial function in helping men to perform sexually, because the nerves involved in erections pass directly alongside the gland; damage to the prostate can have a negative impact on these nerves.

What Can Go Wrong

When things are working normally, the prostate contributes significantly to male health and well-being. But if problems start, this tiny gland can become a source of considerable pain and discomfort.

Prostate diseases are divided into two categories: benign conditions (such as prostate enlargement and inflammation) and more serious conditions such as cancer. Below we'll examine benign prostate diseases and then explain how medical doctors are currently treating them. (Prostate cancer will be discussed more fully in Chapter 8.)

Prostate Enlargement

Approximately one in three men over the age of fifty are believed to have some degree of prostate enlargement. This condition is medically referred to as *benign prostatic hyperplasia,* or *BPH.* ("Hyperplasia" means that there's an abnormal growth of cells and tissues, but because the overgrowth is not cancerous, it's considered *benign.*)

The overgrowth of cells found in BPH is fueled by the male hormone *testosterone* and its by-products. Researchers have found that there are receptor cells on the prostate that attract testosterone molecules. For reasons that aren't entirely clear, prostate cells thrive and grow in the presence of testosterone. (BPH generally becomes worse as men age because their prostates are less able to eradicate the buildup of testosterone.)

Dietary fat, high cholesterol, and nutrient deficiencies can all play a role in causing BPH; in addition, pesticides, food additives, excessive amounts of alcohol, and other toxic chemicals are considered to be contributing factors.

Certain medications that contain antihistamines are also linked to prostate disease. For this reason, men who are being evaluated for BPH or suspect they might have it should *never* take over-the-counter medications without first consulting a doctor.

Symptoms of BPH

Frequent urination (not related to excessive drinking, diseases such as diabetes, or changes in your daily routine); urgency (the feeling that you have to pass urine often); getting up to urinate several times during the night; difficulty or delay in starting urination; incomplete emptying (feeling that there's more urine left after you've finished); dribbling; and a burning sensation are all symptoms of BPH. In some cases, painful ejaculation and problems achieving erections are also symptoms.

Any one or more of the above symptoms should prompt a visit to your physician without delay. In many cases, these symptoms will not mean that anything is seriously wrong, but they *can* suggest the possibility of cancer. (Even if cancer isn't the cause of your symptoms, incomplete passing of urine is potentially dangerous and requires treatment because it can lead to bladder and urinary tract infections as well as kidney problems.)

But even in the absence of symptoms, an annual physical is recommended—especially if you are forty or older.

Your physical should include a careful screening of your prostate by rectal examination (*anal-digital examination*) and by a *PSA* (*prostate-specific antigen*) test.

The rectal examination allows your physician to feel your prostate directly and check for any abnormalities. The PSA is used to check whether a special protein made by your prostate is at above-normal levels; when elevated, the PSA is indicative of but doesn't prove the presence of cancer. (The PSA and other diagnostic tests for the prostate will be discussed more fully in Chapter 8.)

The Standard Treatments for BPH

A number of procedures (and some new medications) are currently being used to treat BPH. One of the most popular treatments is known as **TURP** (*transurethral resection of the prostate*). Developed during the 1950s, TURP has become the gold standard of treatment for prostate enlargement.

TURP is performed in the hospital and usually involves a short-stay visit. The procedure is done under either *general* anesthesia (in which the patient is made to become unconscious) or *spinal* anesthesia (in which the nerves below the waist are temporarily numbed but the patient remains awake).

Once anesthesia takes effect, the urologist inserts a tube-like instrument (called a *resectoscope*) into the penis, through the urethra and into the prostate. The outer tube of the resectoscope remains stationary. Inside it is a smaller tube that has a lens and a wire loop at the end of it. This smaller tube allows the physician to locate the area of the prostate that's enlarged, and will also be used to shave off and cauterize pieces of enlarged prostate tissues.

After the enlarged tissues are found, the doctor moves the small tube in a back-and-forth motion, shaving the tissues with the small wire loop. The entire procedure takes about one hour.

Complications Associated with **TURP**

TURP is generally uneventful, but there can be occasional side effects. For example, the fluids that are used to irrigate (or wash) the area that's being cauterized can cause reactions in some men (including nausea, vomiting, and heart irregularities). Some men also experience retrograde ejaculation (the passage of sperm through the bladder and out into the urine) after leaving the hospital. In a small percentage of men impotence can occur, but this is usually temporary.

In an attempt to minimize these complications, urologists

are developing newer procedures modeled after the TURP. Procedures now under investigation include:

- **Transurethral incision of the prostate** (TUIP). As in a TURP, the doctor enters the prostate with a resectoscope. But instead of trimming the area *inside* the prostatic urethra, the doctor tries to separate the urethra from the enlarged tissues surrounding it, thus allowing urine to flow more easily. Considered a relatively quick and safe procedure, the TUIP can still cause retrograde ejaculation and other side effects similar to those resulting from a TURP.

- **Transurethral needle ablation of the prostate** (TUNA). A special catheterlike probe is placed into the penis, and special needles are then inserted into overgrown prostate tissues. The doctor then discharges bursts of ultrasound energy through the needles, destroying enlarged tissues. Some experts consider TUNA a quicker and safer treatment than either TUIP or TURP, but results are still being evaluated.

- **Transurethral balloon dilatation** (TUBD). A catheter is inserted into the prostatic urethra, and then a balloon is inflated, pressing against the swollen tissues. Proponents of this procedure believe that it effectively opens up the urinary passage. Although considered safer than the TURP and other invasive methods, the TUBD has gotten mixed reviews and is showing variable results. However, some physicians feel that it may be appropriate for younger men not wanting to risk sexual complications such as impotence or for older men not healthy enough to undergo more invasive procedures.

ADDITIONAL THERAPIES FOR BPH

Heat and *laser* treatments are also being investigated for the treatment of BPH. One procedure known as **TUMT** (*transurethral microwave thermotherapy*) involves delivering bursts of heat energy to swollen prostate tissues. Responses are said to be good for some men.

TULIP (*transurethral laser-induced prostatectomy*) and **VLAP** (*visual laser ablation of the prostate*) attempt to reduce BPH via laser probes; however, for some men side effects can equal those of TURP and other standard procedures.

Doctors are also beginning to treat BPH with a new class of drugs. Unfortunately, drug therapies haven't yet replaced TURP and other invasive techniques, but it is hoped they will one day offer prostate patients an option.

Two classes of drugs commonly used for BPH are *alpha blockers* and *androgen-suppressing* agents. Alpha blockers (usually prescribed for high blood pressure) are believed to relax the tissues within the prostate, thereby reducing swelling. Usually alpha blockers are prescribed only to men who have BPH *in addition to* high blood pressure.

Androgen-suppressing drugs interfere with the production of testosterone (linked to abnormal prostate growth).

Among the most common alpha blockers and androgen-suppressing agents on the market are **Hytrin** and **Proscar,** respectively. Despite fairly good results, these drugs are not entirely effective, and they can cause a number of side effects. For example, dizziness, fainting spells, palpitations, nausea, and blurred vision have all been associated with Hytrin therapy. And Proscar has been known to cause decreased sex drive, impotence, and false PSA readings (see Chapter 8 for more on PSA testing).

Prostate Inflammation

Medically referred to as *prostatitis,* inflammation of the prostate is often caused by infectious bacteria such as *Escherichia coli* and *Klebsiella.* Prostate infections can be acquired in a number of ways. Men engaging in unprotected anal intercourse (as nonpassive partners), men who have recurring infections of the bladder or urinary tract such as *cystitis* and *urethritis* (respectively), and men who have undergone invasive procedures to examine their prostates or urinary bladders are at increased risk.

SYMPTOMS OF PROSTATITIS

Prostatitis is divided into two types, *chronic* and *acute.* Both forms can cause symptoms similar to those of BPH, including frequent urination (with or without a burning sensation); painful ejaculation; a feeling of incomplete emptying; and pain in the lower back, in the scrotal area, and around the perineum (the area between the testicles and the rectum). These symptoms tend to come and go with chronic prostatitis, but in the acute form there can be sudden fever, chills, nausea, sweating, and flulike symptoms, as well as more severe pain.

Any or all of the above symptoms should prompt a visit to your doctor or local emergency room clinic without delay.

THE STANDARD TREATMENTS FOR PROSTATITIS

The proper choice of antibiotics is the mainstay of treatment. After examining samples of urine and prostatic fluid, the physician can determine which (if any) bacteria are causing the infection. The correct antibiotic is then prescribed.

Among the more common medicines used for prostatitis are *synthetic penicillins, Bactrim,* and *E-Mycin.* Each of these drugs can have potentially serious side effects and should be prescribed only after a careful history is taken and after all questions pertaining to possible or known drug allergies are carefully answered. Men undergoing antibiotic therapy should always remain under close medical supervision.

Unfortunately from a treatment standpoint, not all cases of prostatitis have a known bacterial cause. For example, *nonbacterial prostatitis* behaves like an infection, but upon examination there is no known bacterium that can be found. Some physicians will still prescribe different types of antibiotics until the right drug match is found and positive results are seen. But other experts are opposed to this practice, claiming that antibiotics not only are potentially dangerous but can lead to drug resistance and further problems later on.

Still another group of doctors believes in "watchful waiting," in which patients receive *no treatment* at all but are observed to see if symptoms become worse.

Cancer of the Prostate

Prostate cancer is believed to be caused by genetic mutations, exposure to cancer-causing chemicals and hormones (such as testosterone), and dietary factors (such as too high a consumption of saturated fat).

Surgery and hormone and radiation therapies are the usual treatments of choice for prostate cancer. These methods (along with the use of natural medicines) will be discussed more fully in Chapters 8 and 9).

CHAPTER TWO

Vitamins, Minerals, and Other Supplements

Nutrition experts have long known that zinc plays an important role in keeping the prostate healthy. In fact, a number of research studies conducted during the last two decades have conclusively shown that zinc inhibits certain enzymes and hormones that are known to cause prostate enlargement. In addition to zinc, other nutrients—including vitamin B_6, fish oil, and amino acids—are also being found to have therapeutic value for the prostate.

Indeed, there are a number of natural substances that can offer your prostate considerable health benefits. But which of these should you take? Equally important, how should you take them, and what side effects, if any, are you to be concerned about?

In this chapter we'll carefully address each of these important issues and provide you with a complete description of key nutrients for your prostate, followed by food sources, suggested dosages, and safety recommendations. At the end of the chapter we'll include suggestions on where and how to buy supplements. In Appendix 1, a complete nutrient regimen tailored for various prostate conditions will be included.

A Balanced Diet Isn't Enough

As you might already suspect, eating a ''balanced diet'' may not be enough to protect your prostate from disease or overcome a disease once it has begun. For example, you might do fine by eating foods rich in zinc and other essential vitamins and minerals—*if* you had a healthy prostate. But the amount of zinc contained in these foods would probably have little *therapeutic* effect if your prostate was enlarged.

In fact, given all the unhealthy conditions men face every day such as stress, aging, and exposure to environmental toxins and pollutants, it is more than likely that many are actually *deficient* in zinc and other prostate-benefiting substances—in spite of a healthy diet. For this reason, naturopathic physicians recommend therapeutic dosages of vitamins, minerals, and other nutrient supplements in the treatment and prevention of prostate diseases.

You can begin planning your own program for a healthier prostate by following the specific nutrient recommendations outlined in this chapter. But before you begin, you'll need to understand the dose equivalents commonly used to describe nutrients.

Understanding Dose Equivalents

Natural medicines for the prostate (as discussed in this chapter and elsewhere) are commonly measured in *grams* (g), *milligrams* (mg), or *micrograms* (mcg). *International units* (IU) are also used.

Micrograms are the smallest measurement used when

describing nutrients, followed by milligrams, and then grams. Technically speaking, one microgram is _one thousandth_ of a milligram, and one milligram is _one thousandth_ of a gram (see **Figure 1**).

Milligrams are typically used for the water-soluble vitamins B and C, and for minerals such as zinc, calcium, and magnesium. Sometimes micrograms are used (as when describing folic acid and selenium). International units are used to describe the oil-soluble vitamins A, D, and E.

The following chart shows the relationship between the different dosage measurements:

FIGURE 1

1,000 micrograms (1,000 mcg)	=	1 milligram (1 mg)
1,000 milligrams (1,000 mg)	=	1 gram (1 g)
10,000 milligrams (10,000 mg)	=	10 grams (10 g)
3 milligrams (3 mg)	=	5,000 international units (5,000 IU)
30 milligrams (30 mg)	=	50,000 international units (50,000 IU)

Nutrients and Other Supplements for the Prostate

ZINC

Zinc is considered among the most important natural medicines for the prostate.

Initially, claims of success for this mineral were based on anecdotal evidence. (_Anecdotal_ means that beneficial reports for a certain medicine or treatment are based not on hard scientific facts but on the personal claims made by individuals.) However, clinically controlled studies have established zinc's usefulness in the treatment of prostate disease. In a landmark study conducted in 1976, for example, researchers found that zinc was able to reduce the swelling and symptoms associated with BPH; they also discovered a parallel between zinc deficiencies in older men and a greater risk for prostate disease.

In a more recent study, researchers also found that zinc reduces prostate enlargement. But perhaps more significant, they found that zinc can actually *lower* harmful testosterone levels in the prostate. As explained in Chapter 1, testosterone is a contributing factor in causing BPH.

Normally testosterone serves a number of valuable functions; it helps boys grow into adult men, makes sexual reproduction possible, and even contributes to healthy levels of aggression. However, testosterone can undergo changes in the body (especially during the fifth and sixth decades of life) and be converted into an unhealthy by-product known as *DT* (or *dihydrotestosterone*). When DT binds with prostate cells, this can lead to an overgrowth of tissues, resulting in BPH.

In order for testosterone to be converted into DT, a special enzyme known as *5-alpha reductase* must be present. But the latest research shows that zinc inhibits 5-alpha reductase—leading to a reduction in prostate size. In addition, zinc gets in the way of DT as it tries to bind with prostate cells, and this causes the DT to be excreted out of the prostate instead of causing damage to it.

Zinc has also been found to inhibit the effects of a hormone known as *prolactin*. Secreted by the pituitary gland, prolactin can be damaging to prostate tissues.

OTHER BENEFITS OF ZINC

Men who take zinc for prostate problems can receive an added bonus: this mineral is also important for faster wound healing, a healthy immune system, and even possible resistance to cancer. (Zinc deficiencies have been linked to a lowered T cell count and reduced disease-fighting ability.) But zinc can also *weaken* disease-fighting immunity when taken in toxic amounts and for long periods of time. In rarer instances, zinc has also been known to *promote* bacterial infections. However, these side effects can be avoided by carefully following the dosage suggestions given below.

GOOD FOOD SOURCES

Pumpkin seeds ($1/4$–$1/2$ cup daily), wheat germ, oatmeal, nuts, oysters, clams, beef, liver, chicken, carrots, peas, brewer's yeast, spinach, and mushrooms are all zinc-rich food sources.

RECOMMENDED DOSAGES

For healthy men over the age of forty, 15 to 30 milligrams of zinc (once daily) is the usual recommended amount. This dosage can be temporarily increased to 90 to 120 milligrams daily for a period of *one month* if you've been diagnosed with BPH or prostatitis. The dosage can then be scaled down to 60 milligrams daily until symptoms improve.

THE BEST FORMS OF ZINC TO TAKE

In order for zinc to be broken down in the intestinal tract, a special chemical known as *picolinic acid* must be present in large enough amounts. But as men become older, their levels of picolinic acid decrease, and this makes zinc absorption more difficult.

To overcome this problem, men who are middle-aged or older should take either *zinc picolinate* or *zinc citrate;* both of these forms of zinc are more readily absorbed by the small intestine—even when picolinic acid levels are low.

SIDE EFFECTS

Zinc can be toxic when taken in doses exceeding *200 milligrams* daily for long periods of time (several months or longer). Signs of toxicity include vomiting and stomach irritation. The suggested therapeutic dose range of 90 to 120 milligrams for one month is not considered toxic— provided the following suggestions are carefully observed:

- Only *chelated* forms of zinc (*zinc picolinate* or *zinc citrate*) should be taken; these tend to be absorbed more fully without creating imbalances of other nutrients, such as copper or selenium.
- Men suffering from viral infections such as a cold or influenza should take lower doses of zinc (not higher than 60 mg).
- If the immune system is actually *impaired* (by a low white blood cell count, AIDS, bone-marrow suppression from chemotherapy, etc.), then it may not be a good idea to supplement with zinc until the problem has been corrected, or unless otherwise directed by a physician.

THE B VITAMINS

Vitamins B_1, B_2, B_3, B_5, B_6, and B_{12} and folic acid (all of which make up the B vitamins) serve a number of important functions relating to health and well-being. But the star among them when it comes to your prostate is **vitamin B_6** (pyridoxine hydrochloride).

As explained earlier, zinc works best when there are adequate amounts of picolinic acid in the intestine. But in order for zinc and picolinic acid to work together, vitamin B_6 must also be present. That's why many experts recommend taking zinc *with* vitamin B_6. This combination may work best when taken separately from other vitamins and minerals (see Appendix 1 for a full supplementation program).

The remaining B vitamins are not as crucial to your prostate but still play useful roles in helping your immune system and possibly your body's ability to inhibit cancer cells.

GOOD FOOD SOURCES

Foods rich in vitamin B_6 include lima beans, soybeans, poultry, tuna, veal, salmon, brewer's yeast, nuts, and avocados. Foods rich in the other B vitamins include blackstrap molasses, beans, brewer's yeast, green leafy vegetables, wheat germ, whole grains, organ meats, milk, cheese, and eggs.

VITAMIN B DEFICIENCIES

You might be eating a well-balanced diet and still experience low levels of vitamin B_6. For example, certain antibiotics (which you may be taking for a prostate infection), diuretics (for weight loss or edema), and alcohol (which should be totally avoided during bouts of BPH or prostatitis) can all deplete your body of B vitamins.

RECOMMENDED DOSAGES

A good daily dose range for vitamin B_6 is 100 milligrams during the first month of treatment for benign prostate disease, followed by 25 to 50 milligrams daily thereafter.

Caution: Taking vitamin B_6 in doses exceeding 200 milligrams daily for several months can result in nervous-system toxicity. If you have any history of neurological disease, consult a physician before taking B$_6$.

ESSENTIAL FATTY ACIDS (EFAs)

Also known as *omega-3 fatty acids,* EFAs are believed to play an important role in maintaining a healthy prostate and also in repairing diseased tissues.

EFAs (which are found in a variety of fish and vegetable oils) are converted into chemical substances in the body known as prostaglandins. Prostaglandins act as chemical messengers that can help turn off undesirable states such as inflammation—often a component of prostate disease. (In some cases unhealthy prostaglandins can actually provoke inflammation; these prostaglandins result from an unhealthy diet, and this issue will be examined more carefully in Chapter 5.)

Clinical trials have established the value of EFAs in the treatment of prostate disease. For example, in one major study conducted at the Lee Foundation for Nutritional Research in Milwaukee, the following benefits were noted from EFA therapy:

- All nineteen study patients with BPH were able to more completely empty their bladders after urination, despite "significant prostatic enlargement."
- Sixty-three percent of the patients were able to fully empty their bladders after several weeks of therapy.
- The majority experienced overall improvement of BPH symptoms.

Additional studies confirmed the Lee Foundation results, and today EFAs are considered an important adjunct in the treatment of prostate disorders.

GOOD FOOD SOURCES

Essential fatty acids are found in vegetable oils (flaxseed or linseed oils), soybeans, anchovies, catfish, herring, freshwater trout, mackerel, mullet, salmon, sardines, and shellfish. Generally the "fattier" the fish, the higher the essential fatty acids. Eating several helpings of fatty fish per week will supply you with adequate amounts of EFAs.

If eating fish isn't to your liking, try taking fish oil capsules; these are sold in most health-food stores or pharmacies. You can also get an adequate amount of essential fatty acids by supplementing with **flaxseed** or **linseed oil** (see supplement recommendations below).

RECOMMENDED DOSAGES

Fish oil supplements can supply you with therapeutic amounts of EFAs. Many of the supplements now available contain 180 milligrams of *EPA* (an omega-3-rich substance) and 120 milligrams of *DHA* (another omega-3-rich substance). A typical daily dosage is 2 fish oil capsules with each meal (for a total of 6 capsules per day).

Some commercial products combine fish oil with *linoleic acid* (another type of EFA), and these are also considered rich sources of omega-3 fatty acids. Generally linoleic acid and fish oil work best in a 1:4 ratio (respectively). See labeling recommendations for dosage.

You can also receive an adequate amount of EFAs by taking 2 tablespoons of *flaxseed* or *linseed oil* daily. **Important note:** Flaxseed or linseed oils are highly unstable and can become rancid very quickly. They should always be kept in a tightly closed bottle, refrigerated immediately after use, and not kept more than one or two months.

SIDE EFFECTS

EFAs are for the most part nontoxic, but mild side effects have been reported after taking large amounts. Depending on your source of EFAs, side effects may include fishy aftertaste, diarrhea, and heartburn. Blood sugar problems and difficulties with blood clotting have also been reported in rare instances. Because of these potential side effects, people who have a family history of stroke, diabetics, or people who are on blood-thinning medications (including aspirin) should check with a physician or naturopathic doctor before taking EFAs.

AMINO ACIDS

Amino acids are not considered frontline therapies for the prostate, but they are believed to help reduce symptoms of BPH and nonbacterial prostatitis, as well as inhibit some of the causes of these disorders. Amino acids can also help lessen the pain associated with prostate inflammation and related urinary-tract infections.

There are twenty-five amino acids in all, and many of these have been found to have a number of therapeutic uses. With regard to prostate disease, *glutamic acid, glycine,* and *alanine* are considered the most beneficial. (*Phenylalanine* is also useful because of its ability to reduce the pain that sometimes accompanies prostate disease.)

HOW THEY WORK

Glutamic acid inhibits the production of prolactin (earlier in the chapter we discussed how prolactin is injurious to prostate tissues). Glycine is also an inhibitor of prolactin and a promoter of tissue healing. Because it is found in high concentrations in the prostate, glycine may have additional importance in the treatment of prostate disorders.

Both glutamic acid and glycine function best when combined with alanine.

Phenylalanine reduces pain by increasing endorphin levels in the brain. (Endorphins are natural morphinelike chemicals that block the brain's sensitivity to pain.) You might wish to try phenylalanine as a nondrug substitute during acute bouts of BPH or prostatitis.

AMINO ACIDS IN THE TREATMENT OF BPH

In one important double-blind study, forty-five men with BPH were treated with a combination of glutamic acid, glycine, and alanine. After two months of therapy, researchers noted the following results:

- Nighttime urination was either relieved or reduced in 95 percent of the patients treated.
- Delayed urination was relieved in 70 percent of the patients.
- Frequency of urination improved in 73 percent of the patients.

Other clinical trials involving glutamic acid, glycine, and alanine have shown similar improvements for men with BPH.

FOOD SOURCES

Brewer's yeast, lean meats, fish, dairy products (skim milk, low-fat yogurt, low-fat cottage cheese), eggs, soybeans, lentils, nuts, and other legumes are all good food sources for amino acids. However, it might be necessary to take amino acid supplements to obtain therapeutic amounts.

RECOMMENDED DOSAGES

The following amino acid dosages are suggested for men with prostatic enlargement or inflammation of the prostate:

Amino Acid	Dosage
*L-glutamic acid	250 mg three times daily
L-glycine	250 mg three times daily
L-alanine	250 mg three times daily

*Amino acids are usually divided into 3 forms: *L, D,* and *DL.* Most amino acids found in the plant and animal kingdoms are of the L variety. For this reason, some experts believe the L forms of glutamic acid, glycine, and alanine to be the most effective for humans.

The following dosage schedule is suggested for men with pain associated with prostatic enlargement or inflammation:

Amino Acid	Dosage
*DL-phenylalanine	250 mg one to three times daily

*The DL form of phenylalanine may offer more pain-reducing benefits than the L or D versions.

SIDE EFFECTS

Glutamic acid, glycine, and alanine are relatively safe in the prescribed amounts. However, the following precautions apply to phenylalanine:

- Any persons who have the rare birth disorder known as *phenylketonuria* should **NOT** take phenylalanine.
- Phenylalanine can sometimes cause headache, a feeling of being ''spaced out,'' or in some instances aggres-

sion. Always assess your response while taking this substance, and if you note any of the above symptoms, reduce the dosage or discontinue altogether.

- It's best *not* to take phenylalanine in the evening (because it may lead to insomnia). It's also best to increase the dosage gradually (in increments of 250 mg over a period of several days).

Other Important Nutrients for the Prostate

Antioxidant vitamins and minerals may all play important roles in the management of prostate problems by a) helping to detoxify toxic chemicals and free radicals in the body that can injure the prostate; b) strengthening the immune system; and c) regulating harmful stress hormones.

Below is a brief listing of helpful antioxidants for your prostate (for additional information and suggestions, see Appendix 1).

Vitamin A (in the form of beta-carotene): Vitamin A and beta-carotene are chemically related substances that can help the body's immune system, prevent the growth of cancer, and also reverse the effects of free radicals potentially harmful to the prostate. It's best to supplement with beta-carotene instead of vitamin A because vitamin A is potentially toxic. An added advantage of taking beta-carotene is that it is converted into vitamin A in the body *as needed*. **Recommended dosages** are between 15,000 and 30,000 IU (10–20 mg) daily. **Side effects** can include a discoloration of the skin, but this harmless condition is *not* a result of the liver damage associated with vitamin A toxicity.

Vitamin C: By helping the body to fight infections associated with the prostate (and also because of its potent free-radical-fighting activity), vitamin C can play an important part in prostate health. **Recommended dosages** are 500 milligrams or more daily in the form of *ascorbic acid* tablets or capsules. The optimum dosage of vitamin C should be determined by what's commonly referred to as bowel tolerance. **Side effects** such as gas and diarrhea usually occur after bowel tolerance has been reached (see Appendix 1 for more details).

Vitamin E (alpha-tocopherol): Besides its antioxidant and free-radical-fighting properties, vitamin E also improves immune-system function. **Recommended doses** are between 200 and 400 IU daily in the form of **d-alpha-tocopherol. Caution:** Some people have transient increases in blood pressure after taking vitamin E supplements. If you suffer from high blood pressure or are concerned about it, consult your physician before taking vitamin E. He or she will probably suggest taking the vitamin in dosages of 100 IU daily and gradually working up to your desired range while periodically checking your blood pressure.

Selenium: This mineral is also known for its powerful antioxidant and anticancer effects. In addition, selenium enhances the effects of vitamin E and for this reason should be taken together with the vitamin. **Recommended dosages** of selenium are 150 to 250 micrograms daily. **Caution:** The mineral can be toxic in doses higher than 300 micrograms. Generally, the **organic form** of selenium is considered safer and less toxic than inorganic forms such as **sodium selenite.**

Additional Detoxifying Minerals

Calcium, magnesium, and *germanium* are also considered important for helping the body to detoxify and eliminate harmful chemicals, pollutants, and other toxic substances that might injure the prostate. See Appendix 1 for recommended dosages and cautions associated with these minerals.

How to Buy and Use Supplements

It is best to purchase supplements that do not contain "incipient fillers" such as yeast, sugars, and coloring. Any one of these additives can cause allergic reactions and mask the otherwise beneficial effects of the nutrient being taken.

While natural vitamins are preferable, many synthetic versions are also acceptable as long as purity and potency are assured. In this regard, it might be wise to choose a name-brand supplement instead of opting for a generic or relatively unknown brand that costs less. Check with your local health food store or supermarket pharmacy.

If you suspect that you do have a deficiency involving any of the nutrients discussed, seek a qualified health professional who can perform the necessary blood and hair analysis to determine your nutritional status.

CHAPTER THREE

Herb and Plant Remedies

Herbs and plants have been used in the treatment of disease for thousands of years. Medical historians tell us that the ancient Egyptians, Indians, and Chinese extensively used herbal remedies for a wide variety of disorders, including those affecting the prostate. In fact, historical records dating from 3000 B.C. show that Chinese physicians routinely used herbs for urinary frequency and other prostate-related symptoms.

Herbal medicine is one of the most popular forms of natural medicine today. Recent polls show, for example, that people are increasingly turning to herbs for the relief of many acute and chronic conditions. And it appears this interest is well grounded, because scientific evidence is now validating the many benefits of herbal medicine. (In this chapter we will review important research studies for each of the single herbs described.)

About This Chapter

If you are suffering from benign prostate disease, certain herbs can help you considerably. In this chapter we're going to look at the most important of these, including *saw palmetto, African pygeum, nettle,* and *bee pollen* (traditionally used in America, Europe, and other Western countries).

We'll also explain the benefits of the more popular herbs from the Far East (as used in traditional Chinese medicine), including *astragalus root, magnolia bark, cinnamon twig, rehmannia,* and *Chinese yam.*

(In Chapter 9 we'll also examine special herbs that can be used as supplements in the treatment of prostate cancer.)

How to Purchase, Prepare, and Use Herbs

Before we examine prostate-healing herbs in more detail, let's first look at how they are prepared and how they are generally used.

Many of the herbs discussed in this chapter are available as *capsules* or *liquids.* Herbs are also available in *loose* or *powdered* form. You can purchase herbs at health food stores, in Chinese markets, or at shops specializing in herbal products. Be sure that the herbs you purchase are guaranteed for potency. Raw, unbottled herbs (which are sold in loose form) are best protected from sunlight and should not be stored in clear plastic bags.

Traditionally, the best forms in which to use herbs so that their true medicinal properties will be activated are as follows:

Decoctions: The hardiest parts of the herb, including its roots and bark, are boiled in water for ten minutes and then allowed to steep. One ounce of herbal material is added to four cups of water. If more than one herb is being used, the sum of the herbs should still equal one ounce. After straining the decoction, you drink it like a tea.

Infusions: Boiling water is poured over the petals, flowers, or leaves of an herb, which then steep for twenty or more minutes. After straining the infusion, you drink it.

Tinctures: Alcohol is used to extract the medicinal properties of an herb. One ounce of dried herbal material (or three ounces of fresh herbs) is mixed with five ounces of alcohol (100 proof vodka can be used). This preparation is then kept in a small sterile airtight bottle and allowed to stand for two to six weeks. Usually one or more teaspoons of the tincture are taken daily, unless otherwise prescribed. Tinctures are available at many health food stores.

Extracts: Extracts are prepared like tinctures, except *water* is used as the extraction medium. If you plan on making your own extracts, remember that some herbs are better activated by preparing them in alcohol; if you have any questions on this matter, seek the help of a qualified herbalist, or better yet, purchase your extracts from a reputable health food store.

Capsules: You can usually purchase any herb you wish in capsule form (capsules typically contain a pure concentration of finely ground dried herbs). You can also prepare your own capsules via the following method: Purchase the herbs you'll be using in finely powdered form. Then fill up empty gelatin capsules with this powder. Empty capsules can be purchased through some health food stores, or you can simply buy an inexpensive vitamin supplement such as pantothenic acid and empty out the capsules accordingly. Usually "size 0" refers to small capsules, and "size 00" to larger ones.

Note: Some herbalists feel that capsules don't yield the same healing properties that decoctions, infusions, tinctures, or extracts do. However, many herbal practitioners routinely prescribe capsules and in some cases instruct their patients to make teas out of the constituents.

Herb and Plant Remedies from the West

SAW PALMETTO

In terms of its prostate-healing benefits, *saw palmetto* shares the spotlight with zinc and vitamin B_6; in fact, this native plant from the southeastern United States is considered a potent ally in the treatment of prostate enlargement and its related conditions.

Technically referred to as *Serenoa repens,* saw palmetto has had a long and illustrious history. First used early this century, saw palmetto had achieved popularity for its alleged benefits as an aphrodisiac, a fertility drug, a nerve tonic, and even a substance that could enlarge the breasts! When combined with other herbs, saw palmetto was also said to stimulate appetite, improve digestion, enhance the absorption of nutrients into the small intestine, and even strengthen thyroid function.

While most of these claims are now open to some speculation, double-blind studies are showing saw palmetto's benefits in treating prostate disease. For example, men suffering from BPH have been found to experience noticeable improvement in their symptoms after taking saw palmetto; in addition, other positive effects on the prostate have been noted (we'll examine these a little later).

Initially, American doctors did use saw palmetto for a number of disorders, including urinary frequency and prostatitis. In fact, saw palmetto was so valued as a *drug* that it was officially listed in the two bibles of American medicine—the *U.S. Pharmacopoeia* and the *National Formulary*. However, the FDA later changed the status of saw palmetto to "unproven drug" and removed it from the *National Formulary* in 1950.

Although many mainstream physicians in the United States are not convinced, several well-controlled European studies *do* show many favorable effects from this plant; saw palmetto is also used extensively in Europe and prescribed by medical doctors as a routine treatment for prostate disease.

HOW IT WORKS

In several double-blind trials, saw palmetto was found to cause a "statistically significant" improvement in men suffering from BPH. Additional studies have also shown that saw palmetto inhibits 5-alpha reductase and the production of *dihydrotestosterone*—the unhealthy by-product of testosterone that, as explained in Chapter 2, can cause prostate enlargement. Extracts of saw palmetto have also been found to prevent DT from binding to prostate cells.

While the scientific evidence for saw palmetto is impressive and compelling, many researchers feel that the plant's true benefits are in *suppressing* the symptoms of BPH, as opposed to actually *reversing* the causes of this disorder.

HOW TO TAKE SAW PALMETTO

The components of saw palmetto that benefit the prostate are called *liposterolic extracts,* and they are mainly contained in the plant's *berries*. The berries are also rich in *carotenes, polysaccharides,* and *fatty acids*.

When taking saw palmetto, look for capsules that contain an *85 to 95 percent concentration of liposterolic extract.* An effective dosage for BPH or prostatitis would be **320 milligrams daily.**

Be careful **not** to purchase supplements that list as their prime ingredients only *saw palmetto berries* or *powder;* these supplements may often boast a higher milligram content per capsule but contain less, or none, of the active liposterolic extracts. Always be sure that the liposterolic amount is listed on the label.

Some people take saw palmetto as an **infusion** (usually 1–3 cups daily), as an **extract** (30–60 drops mixed in water or juice daily), or as a **tincture** (1–3 teaspoons three times daily). However, these methods are **not recommended,** because they may not provide the same beneficial liposterolic extracts found in capsule form, as already noted.

SIDE EFFECTS

Saw palmetto is considered a generally safe herb, but the following precautions should be noted:

- Men who are taking prescription medicines for the prostate, or testosterone-blocking drugs, should consult with a health professional before taking saw palmetto.
- Men who are having a PSA test should alert the doctor they are taking saw palmetto or if possible discontinue taking it a week or more prior to testing; saw palmetto may interfere with PSA readings.

AFRICAN PYGEUM

Next on the list of all-important botanicals is African pygeum (commonly referred to as pygeum). First described in the eighteenth century, pygeum is a plant substance derived from the bark of an evergreen tree. It is extensively used in Europe and is now gaining much popularity in the United States as an effective prostate-healing substance.

Well-controlled studies have confirmed the benefits of this herbal medicine.

HOW IT WORKS

Pygeum has been found to contain three substances that improve prostate health. These substances—*phytosterols, pentacyclic triterpenoids,* and *linear alcohols*—do the following:

Phytosterols reduce inflammation in the prostate by influencing the activity of *prostaglandins.* (Prostaglandins can help reduce inflammation but in some cases actually *provoke* it. For this reason, experts distinguish between "good" and "bad" prostaglandins, and phytosterols appear to block the effects of the "bad" kind.)

Pentacyclic triterpenoids fight inflammation in the prostate; they also inhibit the action of enzymes that cause *edema* (swelling caused by water buildup) within the gland.

Linear alcohols lower *cholesterol* levels; cholesterol is considered one factor in prostate enlargement.

CLINICAL TRIALS INVOLVING PYGEUM

In four carefully controlled trials, patients with BPH and/or prostatitis were compared before and after treatment with pygeum. After the conclusion of the trials, the following results were observed:

- In the first trial, 80 percent of patients with BPH showed significant improvement, including the alleviation of most or all of their symptoms.
- In the second trial, nearly half of the men suffering

from prostatitis experienced improvement; positive results were also seen in cases of *dysuria* (i.e., painful or difficult urination).

- The third trial showed clinical improvement in a majority of men with BPH and prostatitis; however, the best results were seen in men whose symptoms were not severe prior to starting therapy.
- In the fourth trial, men whose mean age was seventy and who were considered good candidates for surgical treatment of BPH experienced clinical improvement after taking a pygeum preparation for sixty days.

Among the many symptoms of BPH or prostatitis that responded well to pygeum were *dysuria* (as already noted), *nocturia* (excessive urination at night), *frequency* (passing water excessively), *perineal heaviness* (a feeling of pain or tenderness in and around the perineum), and *residual urine* (incomplete urination; dribbling after going to the bathroom).

HOW TO TAKE PYGEUM

Like saw palmetto, pygeum works best when specific extracts are used. Pygeum extracts are called *sterols,* and they must be used in therapeutic dosages to have any effect. In the four trials we just told you about, optimum results were seen when 200 milligrams of pygeum sterols were given daily. In some cases, patients experienced improvements in sixty days, but in others results were seen only after four months of treatment.

If you are combining pygeum sterols with the other botanicals described in this chapter, a daily dosage of 50 to 100 milligrams is considered adequate.

Note: Sterols come from the *bark* of the pygeum tree, and the labeling should list this fact. Also keep in mind that the amount of pygeum sterols found in supplements can vary considerably. For example, one supplement may contain only 0.5 percent (one half of 1 percent) total sterols, while another may contain 13 percent.

Purchase only supplements that contain the highest percentage of pygeum sterols.

SIDE EFFECTS

Of all the trials conducted on African pygeum, no significant side effects were noted. However, as with any other natural medicine, always follow the prescribed dosages, and be aware of any unusual changes or sensations that may arise.

NETTLE

It may not be as well known as other botanicals, but nettle (sometimes referred to as stinging nettle) is gaining respect for its role in healing prostate disease. Ironically, nettle is much better known for its *sting* than its medicinal properties.

Nettle has long been part of the folklore of Great Britain, where it grows in plentiful supply among the brush and hillsides, and where many an innocent passerby has been "stung" by its leaves.

Beyond the discomforting sting caused by nettle, many intriguing uses for this versatile plant have been claimed over the centuries. For example, two thousand years ago Roman soldiers rubbed nettle on themselves to help stimulate a sensation of warmth during their exodus into the cool climate of England. Many centuries later, Civil War surgeons found that they could stop bleeding by rubbing nettle juice directly on battle wounds. And in our own century, herbalists have faithfully prescribed nettle for a variety of conditions, including asthma, infections, chest congestion, fatigue, and even hair loss.

While some of these claims are open to debate, nettle's potential in the treatment of benign prostate disease *is* gathering scientific support.

HOW IT WORKS

Nettle extracts have been found to contain a rich assortment of important nutrients, including *iron, potassium, sulfur, magnesium, calcium, chlorophyll,* and *vitamins A and C.* All of these can improve overall health—and some specifically prostate health. Sulfur, for example, is a potent detoxifying substance that helps eliminate toxic chemicals from the body (toxins are one factor that injure prostate tissues). Vitamins A and C are powerful antioxidants, and these are necessary for the protection and healing of damaged or inflamed cell membranes, as found in prostate disease.

Nettle is also known to act as a *diuretic* (stimulant of urine flow) and an *anti-inflammatory.* These actions may further explain nettle's positive effects on BPH, prostatitis, and the urinary retention often associated with these conditions.

HOW TO TAKE NETTLE

Nettle is best taken in capsule form—either in combination with other herbs or on its own.

When taking nettle, use only the *standardized extracts* that contain at least **2.5 milligrams of plant silica** per capsule (this is considered the most active constituent of the plant). Recommended dosage is 250 milligrams one to three times daily.

Nettle can also be taken as an **infusion** (1–3 teaspoons of the granulated leaves in 1 cup of boiling water). The infusion is left to steep ten minutes and then drunk 1 tablespoon at a time for a total of 1 to 3 cups' worth per day.

As a **tincture,** 10 to 30 drops (equal to 1–4 milliliters) can be taken daily.

SIDE EFFECTS

If you are using nettle leaves or powders to prepare your own decoctions or infusions, handle the plant with gloves because of its stinging properties. Otherwise, nettle is considered a safe herb.

BEE POLLEN

One of the more intriguing botanicals, bee pollen has been used to treat prostate conditions for nearly half a century.

Collected from the leaves, buds, and bark of trees, bee pollen is a whole food rich in assorted vitamins and minerals, including *amino acids, calcium, carotene, potassium, plant sterols,* and *vitamin C.* The main extract of bee pollen is *propolis.* Bees gather this substance to construct hives and for nourishment. It's the propolis that is believed to be an active ingredient for reducing prostate enlargement.

HOW IT WORKS

Bee pollen extracts reduce *inflammatory states* in the prostate. How this occurs is not entirely clear, but bee pollen contains *plant sterols* and *essential fatty acids,* which, as noted earlier, are beneficial to the prostate. Bee pollen also improves the body's germ-killing ability and may help to reduce infections in the urinary tract.

CLINICAL TRIALS INVOLVING BEE POLLEN

Medical studies have consistently shown that bee pollen is clinically active against prostate disease. (Most of these studies have tested a prescription drug known as *Prostat,* which is made from bee pollen extract.)

The following are among the most important results to date for men who were given Prostat:

- In a trial conducted at China Medical University, sixty-six patients with BPH were treated with Prostat for six months. After three months of therapy, 92 percent of the patients experienced a "statistically significant reduction" in prostate size. In addition, Prostat was said to have a possibly "curative effect" on the underlying causes of benign prostatic hyperplasia. No important side effects were noted.

- In a six-month double-blind study involving ninety patients, Prostat was found to be "78 percent effective" in the treatment of chronic BPH and nonbacterial prostatitis. For 38 percent of the patients, prostate size returned to normal. In no case was therapy discontinued due to adverse effects. The study was reported in the *British Journal of Urology.*

- Another study—also reported in the *British Journal of Urology*—revealed a "statistically significant improvement" in the urinary flow of prostate patients who received Prostat.

- Japanese researchers found that Prostat resulted in a 96 percent improvement of symptoms relating to prostate disease. In addition, 76 percent of the study patients experienced "objective" improvements such as reduction of prostate size and improved urinary flow.

HOW TO TAKE BEE POLLEN

You can talk to your doctor about taking Prostat if you'd like to try a prescription version of bee pollen. However, some doctors emphasize that pure bee pollen extract can be as effective as Prostat—especially when it is combined with the other herbs and botanicals discussed in this chapter.

If you wish to take bee pollen extract in its natural form, we recommend taking supplements that contain a *high concentration of propolis.*

Bee pollen supplements will usually have either "bee pollen" or "propolis" listed on the label. (Products that contain the pure honeylike form of bee pollen are called "royal jelly," and they don't usually list the amount of propolis contained in them; for this reason, we don't recommend taking royal jelly.)

A good dosage of propolis extract is from 50 to 250 milligrams in capsule form daily.

Note: Be sure not to confuse the actual milligrams of propolis with the *total milligrams* listed for each capsule. For example, if a capsule contains 250 milligrams of *bee pollen,* this tells you nothing about the actual amount of propolis that you'll be taking. (Usually the bee pollen/propolis amounts are listed as a ratio—for example, 250:50 mg, which is a 5:1 ratio of bee pollen to propolis.)

SIDE EFFECTS

For *most people,* bee pollen is safe to take. However, in a small percentage (estimated to be 1 in 200 people), allergic reactions **can occur.** If you or a close family member has any history of allergies to pollen, honey, or bee stings, you should **NOT** take bee pollen products. If you do not suffer from any allergies but are still concerned, start taking bee pollen only in small dosages and then gradually increase the amount until optimum dosage has been reached.

If any unusual symptoms such as wheezing, watery eyes, or other discomfort occurs, discontinue immediately and see your doctor.

The drug Prostat is considered nontoxic and doesn't appear to cause allergic reactions or side effects in people.

Herb and Plant Combinations

Ideally, a combination of saw palmetto and the other botanicals we've told you about can provide the best chances of recovery from prostate disease.

Saw palmetto and African pygeum are often combined in capsule form, and occasionally you'll find nettle added. (If a specific herb or plant substance is not included in the supplement that you choose, purchase it separately and in an appropriate dosage.)

Health food stores, larger retail outlets, and pharmacies sell natural prostate medicines that contain one or more herbs. Some prostate medicines also provide essential nutrients such as zinc or vitamin B_6. But when choosing these products, check to see that they contain the recommended amounts of active ingredients (in many cases, nutrient levels are far too low and should be bolstered by additional supplementation).

One of the better combination products available is called Saw Palmetto Formula. It comes in liquid and pill form and is distributed by General Nutrition Company. In addition to saw palmetto, the product contains zinc, nettle extract, and pygeum bark (but not vitamin B_6).

(See Appendix 1 for full nutrient suggestions.)

Herbal Tonics

Many other herbs, such as *gravelroot, uva-ursi,* and *juniper berries,* have been long valued for their positive effects on the prostate and for their ability to revitalize and replenish the body's healing organs. These herbs are typically combined as a formula and referred to as *tonics.*

Because herbal tonics possess antibacterial properties

and also influence kidney and urinary output, herbalists use them to help purge the prostate of infections and inflammation and to improve stagnant urinary flow.

In his best-selling book *The Way of Herbs,* renowned herbalist Michael Tierra describes two tonics that are considered highly useful for prostate diseases. The first tonic is used to help purify the urinary tract and reduce prostate infection; the second tonic improves urinary flow through enlarged prostate tissues by strengthening the kidneys.

PROSTATE TONIC #1

Purchase the following herbs in *finely ground* powdered form:

Herb	Amount
Gravelroot	½ ounce
Uva-ursi	½ ounce
Parsley root	½ ounce
Goldenseal root	½ ounce
Cayenne	½ ounce
Juniper berries	½ ounce
Marshmallow root	½ ounce
Licorice	¼ ounce

Mix the above herbs together and then fill empty gelatin capsules (size 00) with them. Take 2 capsules three times daily.

PROSTATE TONIC #2

Use the roots or bark to prepare the following herbal tonic:

Herb	Amount
Gravelroot	1 part
Uva-ursi	1 part
Echinacea	1 part

Parsley	1 part
Gingerroot	¼ part
Lobelia	¼ part

Prepare a decoction using 1 ounce of the above herbs in a pint of boiling water. Drink 3 or 4 cups daily.

Chinese Herbal Remedies for the Prostate

Of the many countries that practice herbal medicine, China is considered one of the oldest. In fact, China's most current pharmacopoeia of herbal substances dates back 5,000 years and contains a staggering *5,767* medicinal herbs. Moreover, several dozen of these herbs have undergone scientific evaluation and have been found to benefit a number of diseases, including those of the prostate.

WHAT IS CHINESE HERBAL MEDICINE?

For millennia, the Chinese have believed that diseases result from an imbalance between yin and yang—the two opposite but coexistent life forces that govern human beings and the universe. All aspects of life are viewed in either yin or yang terms; for example, femininity, softness, and nurturing are said to be yin qualities, while masculinity, hardness, and physical strength are yang qualities.

According to the Chinese, yin and yang must exist in a state of balance and harmony for health to exist. Consequently, an excess of one can lead to a deficiency of the other, and this imbalance can ultimately lead to disease.

In traditional Chinese medicine, diseases are treated by first determining which yin and yang forces are out of sync in the body and its various organs. Then specific herbs and plants are prescribed to help put those forces back into balance.

Does It Work?

Much of the success attributed to Chinese herbal medicine over the centuries has largely been based on anecdotal evidence. However, a number of research studies are now establishing the therapeutic value of Chinese herbs and plants and justifying their use in the manufacture of dozens of pharmaceutical products. For example, the popular antihistamine drug Sudafed is made from the Chinese *ephedra* plant; *ginseng, ginkgo,* and *astragalus* are a few of the other many popular Chinese herbs valued for their medicinal uses.

How the Chinese View Prostate Diseases

According to traditional Chinese physicians, prostate diseases do not *originate* in that gland. Instead, "imbalances" in related organs such as the kidneys are said to be responsible.

The Chinese believe that the kidneys act as a major influence on the body's organs and glands. When the kidneys are in a state of yin and yang balance, all other organs remain healthy. But when kidney imbalances occur, other organs can become diseased. Most often kidney imbalances are said to be caused by an excess of "kidney yang."

Excess kidney yang causes a poor flow of urine through the prostate, resulting in a "stagnant condition." This leads to "toxicity" and then chronic irritation and inflammation. In addition, kidney yang is said to cause a number of other conditions, including spleen, heart, and lung problems.

Traditional Chinese physicians emphasize that prostate disease can't be corrected unless excess kidney yang—in all its manifestations—is treated.

An example of the traditional Chinese approach to diagnosing and treating prostate disease can be seen in the case history of a patient named Bob.

After suffering from chronic prostatitis for years and failing to receive much benefit from Western medicine, Bob decided to consult a Chinese practitioner. He eventually settled on an acupuncturist who also specialized in traditional Chinese medicine.

The acupuncturist performed a thorough physical examination to determine the extent of Bob's kidney yang and its relationship to his prostate problems. After the exam, it was determined that Bob's kidneys were passing "poor urine" and that this condition caused chronic prostate irritation. Bob had also experienced respiratory problems over the years, unrelated to cigarettes or other obvious factors. According to the acupuncturist, this was a further sign that deficient kidney yang was at work. It was determined that Bob's lungs would also have to be treated to help his prostate.

Treatment involved a combination of herbs that would strengthen Bob's kidneys and urinary flow and also alleviate his respiratory problems. *Plantain seed, cinnamon bark, cork tree bark, eucamia bark, dogwood, goldenlocks tea,* and *walnut* were a few of the herbs prescribed.

After a few weeks of treatment, Bob noticed an improvement in his overall symptoms, and several months later his prostate had returned to normal.

Of course, Bob's story is presented as an illustration and isn't meant to suggest that standard medical treatment be ignored. But Chinese herbs may provide a worthwhile complement to the standard treatments.

CHINESE HERBAL FORMULAS FOR THE PROSTATE

The formulas described below are among the most popular in China for prostate and kidney disorders. These formulas can be tried for the specified symptoms and conditions listed.

Because these formulas have been designed to have a specific effect on the body—according to the laws of traditional Chinese medicine—**they should be taken separately, and not in combination with the Western herbs already discussed.** The formulas should also be given a fair amount of time to work (one or two months is ample). If results aren't noted, then you can consider taking other herbs or herbal combinations.

When taken according to the suggested dosages, Chinese herbs are considered nontoxic.

Name of Formula:	Rehmannia Eight Formula
Chinese Name:	Pa-Wei-Ti-Huang-Wan
Used For:	Kidney infection, BPH, difficult urination, impotence, fatigue, inflammation
Contains:	Rehmannia, pioscorea, cornus, hoelen, moutan, alisma, cinnamon, aconite
How to Use:	See dosage recommendations on the label.
Name of Formula:	16 Herb Combination
Chinese Name:	Qu shi
Used For:	BPH, prostatitis, urinary tract infection, burning during urination, inflammation
Contains:	Stephania root, hoelen plant, morus root bark, chaenomeles fruit, astragalus root,

atractylodes, rhizome, magnolia bark,
polyporus plant, areal peel, akebia stem,
cinnamon twig, pinellia rhizome, ginger
rhizome, citrus peel, licorice root

How to Use: See dosage recommendations on the
label.

Making Your Own Chinese Herbal Decoction

You can prepare your own Chinese prostate formula by
making a decoction of the following herbs:

Herb	Amount
Rehmannia	1 ounce
Chinese yam	$1/2$ ounce
Dogweed tree	$1/2$ ounce
Alisma plantago	$1/3$ ounce
Tuckahoe	$1/3$ ounce
Tree peony	$1/3$ ounce
Cinnamon	$1/6$ ounce
Achyranthes bidentata	$1/2$ ounce
Plantain	$1/2$ ounce
Aconitum	$1/6$ ounce

According to Daniel Reid in *A Handbook of Chinese
Healing Herbs,* the above decoction can be used for symptoms of BPH and prostatitis, including difficult urination
and perineal pain.

Follow the instructions on decoctions noted at the beginning of this chapter, and then drink the above formula as a
tea.

CHAPTER FOUR

Self-treatment with
Homeopathy

Considered one of the oldest systems of medicine in North America, homeopathy is gaining new popularity as an effective treatment for a wide range of medical conditions, including prostate disease.

Homeopathic medicines are nontoxic and very safe to use. For this reason, you can buy the medicines over-the-counter and without medical supervision—provided you follow guidelines carefully. And because of their user-friendliness, you can try different homeopathic medicines until you find the one that works best. Later in the chapter we'll provide complete information on how to accurately select the right homeopathic medicines.

Another unique aspect of homeopathy is that it can safely be practiced with other treatments you may be receiving—including standard medications and the complementary approaches discussed in this book.

One of the main reasons that homeopathic medicines are so safe is that they are taken in extremely small and nontoxic doses. (Homeopathic physicians believe that the smaller the dosage, the stronger and more effective the medicine.) This practice is opposite to that of orthodox medicine, in which large enough doses of a drug must be given so that appropriate chemical changes occur in the body.

In fact, homeopathy's emphasis on taking smaller dosages of medicine appears to explain its excellent safety record—as well as its effectiveness in treating disease.

What Is Homeopathy?

The practice of homeopathy was started by Samuel Hahnemann in the mid eighteenth century. Hahnemann—a noted physician, scholar, and lecturer—was motivated to create a nontoxic system of medicine after becoming disillusioned with many of the standard medical practices of his day, including bloodletting and purging.

The central idea behind homeopathy is a principle known as the Law of Similars. According to this law, disease symptoms can be alleviated by taking an extremely small dosage of medicine that under healthy circumstances would *cause the same symptoms.* For example, if one tablespoon of ipecac causes vomiting in a healthy person, an extremely small dose would block this effect in a person who was nauseous.

As a more relevant example, if potassium dichromate causes burning and pain in the urinary tract and prostate of a healthy person, tiny amounts would reverse those symptoms in persons with certain types of prostate infection.

These contradictory effects are sometimes compared to vaccine treatments, in which germs or viruses are purposely given to a person to protect that person from getting ill. (There are a number of theories that attempt to explain the mysterious effects of homeopathic medicines, and we'll examine a few of these later in the chapter.)

How Homeopathic Medicines Are Made

Plant substances such as *wild hops, marigolds,* and *poison ivy* make up 80 percent of all homeopathic medicines; the rest derive from animal products such as *snake venom* or *insect matter* and from minerals such as *sulfur* and *potassium.* After homeopathic medicines are selected, they are ground up and then mixed with alcohol or water. This basic mixture is commonly referred to as the *mother tincture.*

According to homeopathic measurements, the mother tincture is considered to have the *smallest and weakest* amount of medicine in it. Further, it's not until the mother tincture is diluted that it actually becomes stronger, or in homeopathic language, *potentized.* (This idea contradicts the ''normal'' standards of measurement, which stipulate that the mother tincture should contain the *most* amount of medicine in it before going through the dilution process.)

Homeopathic medicines are labeled according to their potencies, and these usually consist of a number and letter code such as 1X, 2X, 6X, 12X, or 30X. A 1X potency consists of the original mother tincture and is considered to be the weakest of dosages. A 2X potency (which is the mother tincture diluted with 9 parts alcohol or water) is stronger than 1X. As the numbers increase, so do the dilutions and the relative strengths of the medicines.

Homeopathic medicines also consist of ''C'' and sometimes ''M'' potencies, and these are considered much stronger than their X counterparts. For example, a 1C medicine would consist of the mother tincture diluted with *99 parts* alcohol or water and by comparison would be far stronger than a 1X potency.

How They Are Administered

Homeopathic medicines assume different shapes and forms, including *powders, tablets, pills,* and *liquids.*

Powders come in individual wrappings per single-dose portion, and they are placed under the tongue; tablets are very small, and they too are dissolved under the tongue; pills come in the shape of little round pellets, and they dissolve more quickly than tablets; liquids are supplied in dropper bottles and are usually prescribed 3 to 5 drops per dose, on top of the tongue.

How Do They Work?

Homeopathic physicians are still unsure how their medicines work, but a number of theories have been advanced. One theory holds that extremely diluted medicines contain "electromagnetic properties" that are transported through the body's water stores; these properties are then able to stimulate healing in various parts of the body.

Another theory suggests that the body is able to respond to microscopic particles by a process involving "pattern recognition." According to this idea, specific impressions made by tiny particles are identified by immune-system cells and then communicated throughout the entire immune system, promoting a healing response.

As yet, the exact way in which homeopathic medicines work appears to lie beyond our traditional methods of scientific evaluation and understanding. Yet, well-controlled clinical studies clearly show that homeopathy *is* effective.

Homeopathy and Clinical Trials

There has long been debate on whether minuscule amounts of medicine can heal the body—as homeopaths claim. But researchers are finding that such medicines do in fact work.

The following are just a few examples of research studies that establish the value of homeopathic medicines:

- Researchers at the University of Glasgow found that 82 percent of the asthma patients they treated with extremely high dilutions of *house dust mite* material experienced benefit, versus only 38 percent of those patients who received only a placebo.
- Homeopathic medicine resulted in a statistically significant improvement among children suffering from severe diarrhea and chronic ear infections.
- Bleeding time *decreased* while clotting time *increased* among people taking highly diluted dosages of aspirin; such an opposite effect is precisely what one might expect according to the Law of Similars.
- Pigs and cows that were given homeopathic medicines experienced a lower rate of stillbirths and problems associated with delivery compared with untreated animals.

Homeopathy and the Prostate

Clearly homeopathy appears to work for a number of conditions, but what does current research show regarding prostate disease? Several studies have been performed, and the results have been encouraging.

In a recent study that was reported in the *British Homeopathy Journal,* 80 percent of men suffering from BPH experienced significant improvement within the first two months of treatment. In another study, twenty-three of twenty-seven men with prostatitis were relieved of frequent nighttime urination. And homeopathic medicines were also found effective in up to 95 percent of prostate patients experiencing groin and perineal pain.

Starting Your Own Treatment Program

One of the fundamentals of homeopathy is to accurately prescribe medicines according to *precise symptoms*. To ensure such accuracy, homeopaths rely heavily on a patient's medical history and often spend several hours during the interview phase of an examination.

You too can practice accurate self-treatment with homeopathic medicines—provided you pay very careful attention to your own symptoms and then select the medicines specifically recommended for those symptoms.

In the chart below, we've listed a variety of homeopathic medicines and the exact symptoms for which they're prescribed. Read through the symptoms carefully and narrow down those best describing your own condition. You can then select a medicine as indicated.

Before choosing any homeopathic medicines, keep the following important points in mind:

• The following chart is meant to serve as a starting point for self-treatment. It is up to you, your physician, or your natural-medicine practitioner to decide on the most appropriate dosage. Homeopaths do recommend starting with lower potencies such as 3X or 6X when you aren't completely sure about the medicine you should be taking; 12X potencies are recommended when you are fairly confident, and 30X potencies when you are positive. C potencies can also be tried if you're not achieving good results.

- In rare instances homeopathic medicines may *provoke* symptoms while the healing response is beginning to take place. This phenomenon is not considered a side effect of treatment but a sign that healing is beginning to occur. However, any symptoms that are unusual, painful, or unrelated to your original problem should be investigated by a health professional.

- Homeopathic medicines may occasionally cause vague side effects when they are given to a healthy person or to a person taking the wrong medicine. If anything unusual occurs during treatment, try another medicine or consult with a homeopath.

- Treatment is usually given throughout the duration of an illness, and it is discontinued once favorable results are achieved. Read the directions on the medicine bottle for more information.

HOMEOPATHIC MEDICINES FOR THE PROSTATE

Symptoms	Suggested Medicine
Prostatic enlargement with incontinence or dribbling	Aloe[1]
Last phase of urination causes sharp stinging pain in the urethra	Apis mellifica
BPH in the elderly with urinary frequency	Baryta carb

[1] See the guidelines on pages 51–52 for dosage information, or consult with a homeopathic physician.

Pain following urination; incontinence following laughter, coughing, sneezing, etc.	Causticum
BPH; urinary retention and frequency; perineal pain; soreness in prostate region	Chimaphila
BPH; unsteady, difficult urine flow (urine flow stops and starts)	Conium
Constant urge to urinate; difficult urination with dribbling	Digitalis
Pain in prostatic area that becomes worse when walking; pain that extends from prostate to penis; burning after urination	Kali bichromicum
Urine is slow in starting; must strain to start urine flow; back pain occurs before urination; nighttime frequency	Lycopodium
Frequency with pain; urine flow is poor and becomes worse at night	Medorrhinum
Pain after voiding; pain and soreness in the prostate region extending into the bladder or pelvis; pain becomes worse when lying on back	Pulsatilla
BPH with cystitis (urinary-tract infection)	Sabal serrulata

Burning sensation in the urinary tract when *not* voiding; urine flow stops and starts; impotence relating to prostate disease	Staphysagria
Frequency with pain and burning between the rectum and the bladder	Thuja occidentalis

Where to Buy Homeopathic Medicines

Some health food stores carry a large selection of quality homeopathic medicines. If you're unable to locate the specific medicines that you need, try contacting a pharmaceutical company that manufactures homeopathic products. See Appendix 2 for more information.

CHAPTER FIVE

Helping Your Prostate Through Diet

You've probably heard the old saying "Food is your best medicine." In fact, food's powerful effects on longevity, the heart, cancer prevention, and a host of other important health areas have become well known to most of us. But what's not commonly recognized is that food and other dietary factors are also very good medicine for the prostate.

Foods can help the prostate in a number of ways. Besides serving as a valuable source of nutrients, foods also contain special chemicals and substances that reduce inflammation, promote healing, and offer powerful protection against cancer.

Dietary factors such as fat, toxic chemicals, and food additives must also be taken into account in the treatment of prostate disease because these can all lead to enlargement, inflammation, and possibly cancer.

About This Chapter

To examine the many aspects of diet and prostate health, we've divided this chapter into three sections.

In the first section, "General Dietary Guidelines," we will provide useful, commonsense information on *how* to reduce fat, *what* foods to eat, and *how* you can eliminate harmful chemicals and toxins from your body. If you are healthy but are concerned about preventing prostate problems, the General Dietary Guidelines will help ensure optimum health for your prostate, as well as the rest of your body.

The second section, entitled "Special Diets for the Prostate," will examine dietary programs that can be used for specific prostate problems.

Following is a brief summary of each program:

Diet Plan #1 can be used if you are suffering from BPH. This plan emphasizes a more significant reduction in fat and cholesterol, as well as other necessary dietary changes.

Diet Plan #2 is for prostate inflammation and related conditions caused by infection. This program consists of a wholesome diet rich in fruits, vegetables, and juices to help acidify and cleanse the urinary tract.

(Special dietary interventions for prostate cancer will be fully discussed in Chapter 9.)

Finally, in the last section, "Healing Through Fasting," we will provide useful information on how a short-term fast can benefit your prostate.

General Dietary Guidelines

Whether you are healthy, suffer from an enlarged prostate, or are simply concerned about cancer prevention, the most important favor you can do for yourself is to reduce total dietary fat.

Before we make specific recommendations on *how much* fat you should be eating, let's examine a few commonsense guidelines to help you get started cutting down on fat easily and effectively.

GOOD VERSUS BAD FATS

Remember the last time you fried a hamburger or a juicy steak (assuming, that is, that you are not a vegetarian) and then, after enjoying your meal, you let the frying pan sit on the stove for a few hours while you went off to digest your meal? Now recall what happened after the hamburger or steak grease cooled down: It solidified into a gelatinous mass of white gooey stuff that just sat in the pan. Your next problem probably became *how to get rid of this stuff.* You may have even been told by your wife, mother, or the plumber to *never* throw this stuff into the sink, because it might clog the pipes!

Well, it's precisely this same white goo (otherwise known as *saturated fat*) that literally clogs arteries and causes people to suffer heart attacks and other diseases. Equally significant, recent studies are showing a strong link between saturated fat and prostate disease. Saturated fats also possess *carcinogenic, mutagenic,* and *free-radical*-damaging properties. All these conditions lead to abnormal changes in healthy cells, with prostate cancer being one possible result.

Before we condemn fat altogether, it's important to remember that *not all fat is unhealthy.* In fact, your body requires some of it to supply energy and to maintain health. However, it is very important to choose the *right kind* of fat in a program of healthy eating.

According to nutritionists, the healthiest fats are the *monounsaturates* (found in olive and canola oils). *Saturated fats* (found in whole dairy products, hydrogenated oils, red meats, duck, chicken skin, etc.) are considered the worst, so avoid them like the plague.

Interestingly, *polyunsaturated fats* (found in vegetable, corn, soybean, sunflower, and safflower oils, and in margarine) are not good for you—despite all the favorable publicity you may have heard about them. The reason is, polyunsaturates are highly unstable, more prone to oxidation, and more readily capable of forming dangerous free radicals.

Note: Even though they are better for you, monounsaturates, like all oils, are prone to some degree of oxidation when exposed to air or heat for long periods of time. So be sure to always keep your oils refrigerated or in a cool place, and keep bottles tightly closed. Consider buying your oils in aerosol cans that contain added antioxidants; these can protect oils from oxidation.

Since all fats will boost your daily intake of calories and put you at risk for being overweight and unhealthy, keep the following rule in mind:

> **When you do use fats and oils, always choose the healthiest ones and use them *in moderation*—so that your daily calories from fat are not higher than 30 percent of total calorie intake.**

YOUR DAILY CALORIES FROM FAT

While all extra calories contribute to weight gain, it's your *calories from fat* that tend to do so more easily. And with increased weight, there's a greater risk of prostate disease. (Of course, you don't necessarily have to be overweight to develop problems; there are plenty of thin men who have higher-than-average fat intakes—and who also suffer from prostate disease.)

As mentioned earlier, to stay healthy you should not consume more than 30 percent of your daily calories from fat;

according to recent studies, the higher you go above 30 percent, the greater your risk of disease, and the lower you stay below 30 percent, the lower your risk.

By knowing what your average calories-from-fat percentage is, you'll be able to make adjustments in your daily eating habits as required by your medical circumstances (we'll tell you about what adjustments to make a little later).

How to Calculate Your Daily Calories from Fat

One of the best ways to begin cutting down on fat is to see how much of it you actually consume on an average day.

To calculate your daily calories from fat, use the following method:

First keep a diary or journal of your average eating habits for a few days. Next figure out what your average daily calories are, and total the amount of fat grams eaten in one day. (You can read the labels on the foods you eat; these will provide you with all the calorie and fat information you'll need.)

As an example, let's say that on an average day you consume 2,000 calories and 67 fat grams; the following two-step formula will tell you what your percentage of calories from fat is:

1. Multiply the amount of fat grams (67) by the number 9 (9 is always the number used in this formula). $67 \times 9 = 603$.
2. Take the number 603 and calculate what percentage this number is of your total daily calories. To do this, divide 603 by 2,000 ($603 \div 2,000$). The result is 30 percent.

In this example, 30 percent of your daily calories would be from fat (about the average that's recommended from the American Dietetic Association).

Now suppose that you needed to cut your daily fat calories down to 20 percent because of prostate disease; in this case, you would simply have to limit yourself to 44 (instead of 67) fat grams every day to meet this quota.

Use the following chart to quickly determine what your total daily fat grams should be, based on different calories-from-fat percentages:

Your Average Daily Calories	Total Daily Fat Grams at 30% (daily calories from fat)	at 25%	at 20%
1,400	47	39	31
1,600	53	45	36
1,800	60	50	40
2,000	67	56	44
2,200	73	61	49
2,400	80	67	53
2,600	87	72	58

BE CAREFUL OF FOOD LABELS

Instead of counting fat grams, some people read the calories-from-fat percentages listed on food labels to help them choose low-fat products. However, this "information" can be downright confusing. Like most other processed foods, which supply information in the same or similar formats, consider the following example, which appears on a popular peanut butter spread:

Amount Per Serving	% Daily Values*
Total Fat 16 g	25%

An unsuspecting consumer might purchase this product, thinking the total fat content to be 25 percent per serving. But in small print in a lower corner of the label reads the following caveat:

*Percentage Daily Values (PDV) are based on a 2,000-calorie diet and a total of 64 fat grams per day.

Exactly *what* does this mean? A careful reading of the fine print reveals the answer.

The label is actually saying that 16 grams of fat per serving of peanut butter is equivalent to 25 percent of the total "daily values" (i.e., 64 fat grams). But exactly *where* do they get the "daily values" from? From a hypothetical 2,000-calorie/64-fat-gram diet that has absolutely nothing to do with what your diet may really be like.

In reality, the *actual* fat calories in the peanut butter are listed as *150 out of a total 200 per serving,* which translates to a colossal 75 percent fat calories per serving!

You can see why it is so important to read *all the information* listed on labels, and not only those "facts" that the manufacturers want you to read.

Watching the Types of Foods That You Eat

By following a few commonsense rules about the types of foods you should choose every day, you will be guaranteed success in a program of total fat and cholesterol reduction. Being able to spot good from bad food choices will also mean that you won't have to constantly read labels for fat grams or other information.

You can use the United States Department of Agriculture's Food Guide Pyramid to help you make healthy food choices. The food pyramid consists of the following six categories:

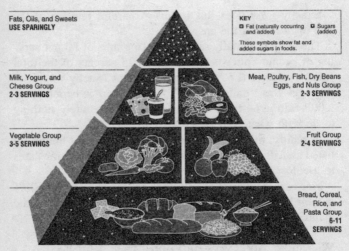

KEY

☐ Fat (naturally occurring and added)   ☐ Sugars (added)

These symbols show fat and added sugars in foods.

Fats, Oils, and Sweets
USE SPARINGLY

Milk, Yogurt, and
Cheese Group
2-3 SERVINGS

Meat, Poultry, Fish, Dry Beans
Eggs, and Nuts Group
2-3 SERVINGS

Vegetable Group
3-5 SERVINGS

Fruit Group
2-4 SERVINGS

Bread, Cereal,
Rice, and
Pasta Group
**6-11
SERVINGS**

Source: U.S. Department of Agriculture/U.S. Department of Human Services

- **Fats, Oils, and Sweets.** Fatty foods should be used very sparingly because they supply lots of calories but few nutrients. The American Dietetic Association recommends limiting the use of sweet salad dressings (to 1 or 2 tablespoons); going easy on spreads, toppings, and sauces; and limiting the amount of cream, cheese, and butter (see below for more specific recommendations).

- **Milk, Yogurt, and Cheese Group.** Two or three servings of milk and foods made from milk (such as low-fat yogurt, feta cheese, fat-free sour cream, and low-fat cream cheese) are recommended daily. A serving is considered to be 1 glass of skim milk, 2 slices of cheese, or 1 cup of yogurt.

- **Meat, Poultry, Fish, Dry Beans, Eggs, and Nuts Group.** Foods in this group include cooked lean meats (such as pork loin), poultry (without the skin), and fish; also included are lentils, peas, baked beans, eggs, and peanut butter. Two or three servings are recommended daily.

  One cup of cooked lentils, 2 eggs, or 4 tablespoons of peanut butter are each considered a serving; 2 to 3 ounces of meat, poultry, or fish is also considered a single serving.

- **Vegetable Group.** Three to five servings of dark green and deep yellow vegetables are recommended. Good vegetable choices include carrots, kale, spinach, brussels sprouts, bell peppers, tomatoes, and green peas. Arugula, chicory, kale, and romaine lettuce are also excellent choices.

  A half cup of chopped vegetables; 1 cup of raw leafy vegetables (lettuce, spinach, etc.); 1/2 cup of cooked vegetables; 1/2 cup of cooked legumes (beans, peas, or lentils); and 1 small baked potato are each considered a vegetable serving.

- **Fruit Group.** Two to four servings daily are recommended. Fruit choices should include the more common (apples, oranges, and bananas) and the less common (kiwifruit, berries, mangosteens, etc.).

  One medium fruit, $1/2$ grapefruit, $3/4$ cup of juice, and $1/2$ cup of berries are each considered a serving.

- **Bread, Cereal, Rice, and Pasta Group.** Six to eleven servings are recommended daily of the following foods: whole-wheat pasta, whole-grain bread, whole-grain cereals, bran flakes, oatmeal, cooked barley, wheat germ, brown rice, bagels, English muffins, buckwheat, and millet. One slice of bread, $1/2$ roll, and $1/2$ cup of cooked rice or pasta are each considered a serving.

Without undermining the importance of the USDA pyramid and the food choices it represents, the following additional guidelines are recommended for maintaining prostate health:

- Avoid processed sugars and overly sweet foods. There is some evidence that excess sugar can lead to the manufacture of *bad prostaglandins*—chemicals that *turn on* inflammatory states in the prostate. (See Chapter 2 for an explanation of prostaglandins.) Choose fructose or turbinado brown sugar instead of white table sugar.

- Avoid foods with saturated or processed fats or oils in them; these include lard, palm oil, and hydrogenated or partially hydrogenated oils. Also avoid processed cheeses; luncheon meats; and enriched, bleached, and refined foods (cakes, breads, pies, etc.).

- Eat at least 2 to 4 helpings weekly of zinc- and EFA-rich foods, including shellfish, cooked oysters, herring, salmon, sardines, whole fish, peas, and carrots. Also eat at least two to four helpings weekly of soy-based foods, including soybeans and soy milk, and organic peanuts.

- Eat at least two portions weekly of tomatoes and tomato-based foods (tomato sauce, stewed or cooked tomatoes, tomato soup, etc.).

- If you drink, limit your amount of alcohol to 1 or 2 ounces of spirits or 1 or 2 glasses of white wine daily. White wine is better than red, and spirits are better than either wine or beer. If possible, avoid beer altogether because many experts consider it one of the worst offenders of the prostate.

- Be sure that your diet contains a generous amount of *detoxifying* foods that contain *sulfur, calcium, magnesium,* the *carotenes,* and *chlorophyll.* Good detoxifying foods include asparagus, broccoli, cabbage, cauliflower, and other cruciferous vegetables; whole seeds; legumes; lentils; garlic; and onions.*

- Avoid fried, sautéed, charcoal broiled, smoked, creamed, buttered, or browned foods. Instead, choose roasted, braised, steamed, baked, poached, or microwaved foods. Barbecued foods are okay—provided that you wrap them up in aluminum foil during cooking. This prevents juices from dropping onto coals and forming benzoapyrenes and other potent carcinogens.

- *Caution:* When eating out at restaurants, request that meals be cooked according to *your preferences.* Also be wary of restaurants that offer ''low-cholesterol''

---

* Because produce is often sprayed with pesticides and other chemicals, consider purchasing your fruits and vegetables directly from greengrocers, farmers, or health food stores that guarantee chemical-free, or organic, products.

fried foods as "healthy" alternatives. Avoid these foods at all costs! While they might be lower in cholesterol, they are still fried (usually in polyunsaturated oils) and therefore highly unstable and loaded with free radicals.

Also be sure to take supplements with your diet. For additional supplement suggestions, see Appendix 1 under "General Supplementation Program for Maintaining Prostate Health."

Special Diets for the Prostate

The following diet plans can be used to treat or prevent specific prostate problems. Select the plan that best fits your needs, then follow the recommendations given.

Keep in mind that there's a certain degree of flexibility within each program. For example, one diet might suggest a daily calories-from-fat intake of 25 to 30 percent daily, but depending on individual factors such as your age, weight, and family history, you might opt for either the higher or the lower end of the percentage range. (We'll include suggestions for helping you to determine what this range should be.)

Caution: Seek additional advice from a medical professional for concerns you may have about following a diet or about what your individual needs might be. Do not begin a dietary program if you haven't yet had a complete medical exam for any symptoms suggestive of BPH or other prostate-related disorders.

Diet Plan #1: For Men with Chronic BPH
• *Don't consume more than 20 percent daily calories from fat.* Try this program for at least several months to determine improvement. (See below for a tasty sample

diet.) You might also wish to try a short fast (see the end of this chapter for complete guidelines).

- Eat at least *four helpings weekly* of zinc- and EFA-rich foods (shellfish, cooked oysters, herring, whole fish, peas, and carrots); eat four to seven helpings weekly of soy-based foods (soybeans, soy paste, soy milk, tofu).
- Consume fiber daily (bran, whole grains, oatmeal, wheat germ, etc., and fruits with the skin on them).
- Try to eat only organic foods—i.e., foods that are not chemically treated (free-range, hormone-free poultry; seven-grain breads; pesticide-free produce, etc., should all be part of your diet).
- Eliminate alcohol, coffee, and tea—especially throughout the duration of your BPH.
- Eliminate hot, spicy foods and any other irritant that can inflame the urinary tract.
- Drink at least eight glasses of *pure* springwater daily.
- Do not take any over-the-counter medications—especially antihistamines—unless under the direction of your doctor.

20 Percent Calories from Fat: Sample Diet
Breakfast
Fresh fruit with skin (apples, pears, nectarines, etc.)
Fat-free yogurt with ½ cup crushed nuts and seeds (pumpkin seeds, sunflower seeds, almonds)
1 slice whole-grain bread with naturally sweetened jam
1 cup herbal tea (chamomile; orange blossom; strawberry leaf, etc.)

Mid-Morning Snack
1 slice whole-grain bread, toasted
1 cup herbal tea

Lunch

1 serving of tuna salad (prepared with 1 tsp. olive oil, chopped onion, parsley, and lemon)

1 baked potato with skin (fat-free yogurt can be added for taste)

tossed salad with zucchini, cucumbers, tomatoes, and fat-free dressing

glass of fat-free chocolate milk or springwater, as desired

Mid-Afternoon Snack

1 glass tomato juice

1 serving of cooked brown rice; 1 tbsp. Parmesan or Romano cheese sprinkled on the rice

Dinner

1 serving of shellfish (boiled lobster, crab legs, etc.), tuna steak, or salmon

Fish can also be prepared by broiling it in garlic and herbs (parsley, oregano, and garlic powder will do). Add a few ounces of water, or 1 teaspoon of olive oil, and several sprinkles of vinegar.

Tossed salad with fat-free dressing

Boiled or baked potatoes

Pure springwater

Before-Bed Snack

One of the following:

Fat-free fudge brownie

Apples stewed in cinnamon and 1 tsp. turbinado sugar

1 small can of fruit cocktail without added sugar

For supplement suggestions, see Appendix 1 under "Supplementation Program for BPH or Nonbacterial Prostatitis."

Diet Plan #2: For Men with Prostate Infections and Related Conditions*

Recommendations:
- Drink plenty of fluids; cranberry juice is highly recommended as a means of acidifying the urine. (Most commercially prepared cranberry juice is too weak to acidify the urinary tract. Health food stores sell the unsweetened version, and this can be made less tart by mixing it with a little apple juice.)
- Drink herbal teas throughout the day to stimulate diuresis (passing of urine). The best herbal diuretics are *juniper, buchu, uva-ursi,* and *corn silk. Celery seed* tea is also considered excellent for its diuretic and anti-inflammatory properties. (See Chapter 3 for more information on herbal tonics for prostate-related infections.)
- Drink herbal teas containing *echinacea* for their immune-enhancing properties.
- Consume foods rich in vitamin C (citrus fruits, fresh-squeezed lemon juice, blueberries, and bananas). Dietary vitamin C is also important for acidifying the urinary tract and for reducing infections. **Caution:** Persons with diverticulitis should avoid any fruits such as blueberries that contain tiny seeds.
- Eat generous helpings of low-fat or fat-free dairy

---

* *Note:* Any infection in the urinary tract such as cystitis or urethritis can directly affect the prostate and can also be helped by the following diet.

products and other calcium-rich foods to reduce bladder irritability.
- Completely avoid coffee, tea, and alcohol.
- If you have concurrent BPH *and* an infection, follow **Diet Plan #1**—in addition to the above suggestions.

For additional supplement suggestions, see Appendix 1 under "Supplementation Program for Prostate Infections and Related Conditions."

Note: If your prostatitis is related to a current kidney infection or if you've developed such an infection as the result of prostatitis or BPH, you've probably been advised to cut down on or avoid some of the foods recommended in this chapter. These include foods high in *oxalates* such as citrus fruits, berries, rhubarb, leafy green vegetables, beets, beans, peppers, parsley, spinach, carrots, cucumbers, and celery.

Oxalate-rich foods are important for your prostate, but you can still choose from a large selection of *nonoxalate* foods as described throughout this chapter. Nonoxalate foods rich in zinc and EFAs include whole fish and shellfish, tomatoes, noncitrus fruits, asparagus, cauliflower, whole seeds, wheat germ, wheat bran, potatoes, whole grains, nuts and seeds, legumes, lentils, garlic, and onions.

Healing Through Fasting

If you've ever owned a dog, a cat, or another domestic animal, recall a time when that animal became sick; chances are, the animal lay down in its favorite corner and *stopped eating* until the crisis passed. We humans also lose our desire to eat during periods of illness, and this is nature's way of preventing food intake and shutting down the digestive process.

Why does nature shut our digestive process down when

we're ill? Because eating puts stress on the major organs of digestion and metabolism, and food abstinence allows those organs a chance to perform other tasks, such as the elimination of toxins from the blood and the body.

The idea of *voluntarily* not eating as a method of healing has been practiced since prebiblical times. In fact, history records many examples of chronic and acute illnesses that responded to fasting—sometimes dramatically.

Today scientific research is substantiating the health benefits of fasting, and the age-old practice is once again becoming popular throughout many parts of the world—including the United States.

FASTING AND DISEASE

According to Dr. Marshall Mandell, one of America's foremost experts on foods, diet, and disease, a number of conditions have been helped by fasting. Mandell explains that some patients suffering with asthma, ulcerative colitis, migraine headaches, depression, and other chronic conditions have reported benefits from fasting.

Natural practitioners have traditionally used fasting in the treatment of prostate diseases such as BPH and prostatitis, and they too have claimed favorable results. According to Dr. Leon Chaitow, a leading naturopathic physician who has treated hundreds of men with prostate disease, fasting creates a period of "physiological rest" that markedly improves the body's chances to heal the prostate.

WHAT HAPPENS DURING A FAST?

When you stop eating for a period of time, a number of metabolic changes take place in your body.

During the first day of a fast, your body consumes its own protein reserves for nourishment. Then, after a day or two, a *protein-sparing* mechanism is switched on, and your body begins to draw on its *fat* reserves. As long as the body uses its own fats, there is no danger of the severe weight loss usually seen in cases of starvation.

Many people confuse fasting with starvation, but the two are completely different phenomena. During a normal fast (which for a *healthy person* can last anywhere from one to five days without any problems), hunger is initially experienced, but as the body's metabolism switches gears and fat reserves are used, the hunger subsides. During starvation, on the other hand, a person becomes severely malnourished after not eating proper foods over a period of many weeks or months. In this case, a severe and constant state of hunger is often experienced.

The fact is, hunger should not be a problem if you are fasting correctly. (A little later we'll provide guidelines on how to conduct a fast safely and how to avoid any possible problems that may arise.)

DIFFERENT TYPES OF FAST

Two common approaches to fasting are the *semifast* (only pure water and unsweetened fruit juices are consumed) and the *total fast* (nothing but water is consumed). Both fasts offer potential advantages and disadvantages.

Some practitioners believe that a semifast doesn't allow the protein-sparing switch to be turned on. When this happens, the body's hunger-control mechanisms are "teased" with hints of food, and a constant state of hunger results. But other experts say that a total fast may be too difficult for some people—especially those who are physically dependent on foods and other addictive substances such as sugar, alcohol, and tobacco.

In view of these potential problems, which fast should you choose? Consider the following guidelines to help you decide:

If you suffer from *food addictions* (sugar, wheat, corn, chocolate, and caffeine are among the most prominent), *chemical addictions* (to nicotine, caffeine, etc.), and *hunger-control problems,* you might want to try a semifast. If you don't suffer from any known food or chemical addictions and you've already been following the diet principles discussed in this chapter, a two- to four-day complete fast shouldn't be a major problem.

Whichever fast you do choose, make sure that you consult with a physician before starting.

Typically, the following criteria should be met before starting a fast:

- You are in generally good health. (Diseases such as cancer, diabetes, hypoglycemia, anemia, kidney or uric-acid diseases, and heart disease usually preclude one from doing a fast.)
- You are not suffering from malnutrition or appetite loss due to disease, and you are not frail or significantly underweight.
- You have ample downtime to relax, and you do not have to do physically hard work while fasting.

STARTING THE FAST

It's usually best to start a fast right before the weekend (or at the end of your workweek). The fewer work distractions and stresses you face, the better.

You can start a semifast by eating a light fruit meal on, say, a Friday night, and then consuming only pure bottled springwater and unsweetened juices throughout the weekend whenever you feel hungry. You can also do a complete fast the same way, but instead of starting with a fruit meal, begin by consuming pure water, and continue to do so throughout the weekend.

It's best to not be around people when they're eating and to avoid tempting images of food (as displayed on television, in magazines, etc.).

You might develop a few symptoms during your fast such as headache, a runny nose, fatigue, a white coating on the tongue, and similar complaints. According to nutrition experts, these symptoms (called *flare-ups*) mean that the body is purging itself of toxins and pollutants. In fact, flare-ups are considered a *good sign* that the fast is working.

What should you do if a flare-up does occur? If it is minor and doesn't become too uncomfortable, then there's no cause for alarm. (In most cases, the symptoms will pass in less than a day.) However, if the symptoms are bothersome, you might want to try one of the following remedies as suggested by Dr. Mandell:

- Take 2 tablespoons of unflavored milk of magnesia at the first sign of symptoms;

  or

- Take 1 heaping teaspoon of 2 parts baking soda and 1 part potassium bicarbonate in a large glass of pure springwater;

  or

- Try Alka-Seltzer Gold.

Dr. Mandell explains that many fast-related symptoms result from a release of acids into the bloodstream, and the above remedies contain salts that displace the acids.

Persons with heart or kidney disease should not take these remedies unless under the advice of a physician.

BREAKING THE FAST
On the day after your fast is completed, begin reintroducing fruits and vegetables (steamed or raw) into your diet,

followed by light foods (cereals, soups, broth, etc.). After a day or two of light meals, regular meals can once again be eaten.

ADDITIONAL RECOMMENDATIONS

The following dos and don'ts will make your fasting experience all the more successful and rewarding:

- Follow one of the diet plans examined in this chapter for at least two weeks before starting the fast. It's easier to do a fast when you've already been on a proper diet.
- Wean off foods and other substances you crave or are addicted to (such as coffee, tea, chocolate, alcohol) before starting your fast.
- Don't begin a fast if you are on medication.
- During a fast, consume 8 to 12 glasses or more of pure bottled springwater daily; it's best to drink water from glass containers or vessels, not plastic or synthetic ones.
- During a complete fast, **NEVER** eat anything—however small it may be; eating can throw a monkey wrench into your body's hunger mechanism and keep you feeling hungry throughout the fast period.
- Try to avoid exposure to chemicals or environmental pollutants during the fast; these include chlorine, aerosol sprays, fluoride (as found in toothpaste), carbon products, and anything else that might compromise your body's detoxification process.
- Discontinue any vitamins you may be taking before starting your fast. If you are taking high doses of vitamin C, discontinue gradually to avoid the ''rebound effect'' (see Appendix 1 for more details).

CHAPTER SIX

Special Exercises, Massage, and Hydrotherapy

In addition to all the natural medicines that work *within* our bodies, there are also therapies for the prostate that are applied *physically,* and these include *special exercises, reflexology,* and *hydrotherapy.*

Physical therapies have indirectly proved quite valuable for BPH, prostatitis, and other disorders of the urinary tract. What's more, they can safely be combined with any of the other therapies you may be receiving.

Because exercise is one of the most familiar and universal forms of physical therapy, we'll begin the chapter by telling you about three specific types that can benefit the prostate and improve related conditions such as prostate enlargement and infection.

Special Exercise #1: Aerobics

The primary goal of aerobics is to achieve peak cardiac output; once peak output is achieved, the blood and oxygen supply to the prostate and other organs also reaches peak efficiency. (This state is ideal for healing and for faster recovery time from disease.) In addition, aerobic exercises can help to stabilize hormones in the body that injure the prostate.

To achieve the benefits of aerobics, most health experts recommend brisk walking or swimming three or four days per week. Exercises that involve bumping or jolting the body (*horseback riding, dirt-bike riding, wrestling,* etc.) **are not** recommended if you have BPH or prostatitis.

Caution: Never exercise in the heat or after a meal, and always make sure that you are fully hydrated several hours before starting.

Finding Your Target Heart Rate

To help you determine how much you should exercise at any given time, use your *target heart rate* as a gauge. The following formula will help you to calculate your target heart rate:

Subtract your age from the number 220. Then calculate what 80 percent of that number is. For example, if you are fifty years old, $220 - 50 = 170$. Eighty percent of 170 is 136. Your target heart rate would thus be 136, and your heart rate *should not exceed* (but should remain at) *136 beats per minute* throughout the duration of your exercise. (Some experts recommend lowering your target rate number by 20 percent until you get used to your exercise program; in the above example, this would be 109.) **Ten to 20 minutes** of peak heart effort is considered adequate for deriving full aerobic benefit.

To keep tabs on your heart rate, gently place your fore-finger (not your thumb) on your carotid artery, located next to the Adam's apple, and count your pulse for a fifteen-second period. Then multiply by 4. That's your pulse per minute. While exercising, periodically monitor your pulse to make sure that you're staying close to or at your target heart rate.

Caution: If any of the following conditions apply to you, **DO NOT** begin a program of aerobic exercise without first consulting a physician:

- You are over fifty and/or overweight.
- You have typically eaten a high-fat, low-fiber diet most of your life.
- You smoke and/or drink alcoholic beverages regularly.
- You lead a sedentary lifestyle and rarely exercise.
- You have a history of heart disease (congenital or acquired) in your family, or you suspect that you may have heart disease.
- You have high blood pressure (even if you don't suspect any problems, you should routinely check your blood pressure; most drugstores and larger supermarkets have do-it-yourself blood pressure testing).
- You tire very easily and become short of breath after only little exertion.
- You experience any other symptoms that are or may be cardiac in origin, such as palpitations, dizziness, or chest pain.

If you have any questions or concerns about your health, always see a physician for a thorough workup before starting aerobics.

Special Exercise #2: Yoga

A form of healing that's been in existence for 5,000 years, yoga is based on the principle that health results from a harmonious balance among mind, body, and spirit.

Yoga, which has been described as "a system of exercising involving postures [and] breathing . . . ," has shown clinical benefits for many acute and chronic medical conditions. For example, yoga has been shown to improve breathing among people with emphysema, prevent pneumonia in the elderly, improve circulation for people with artery disease, and improve eyesight in the visually impaired.

Yoga exercises are also considered highly beneficial for improving circulation to the prostate while decreasing fluid buildup and congestion in that gland.

Yoga Postures for the Prostate

There are several easy-to-use yoga exercises that can benefit your prostate.

Central to each exercise is what's known as a *posture*. The posture is considered a state of dynamic tension in which you are holding your body in a certain position *but not* straining or tensing up your muscles to maintain that position.

The following yoga postures are considered among the most important for the prostate. Try all of them, and then rotate postures for maximum benefit (i.e., do one on the first day, another on the second day, etc.).

- **Cobra Posture:** Lie flat on your stomach. Place your hands palms down so that your elbows are bent and your hands are tucked under your shoulders. (Your elbows should not be pointed sideways.) Take in a deep, slow breath, and while doing so, curl your eyes and head back as far as they will go (without straining them); then lift your chest and stomach up slowly (while arching your back inward). At this point, your hipbones should remain on the floor, and your arms should be slightly bent (see **Figure 1**). Maintain this position for a few seconds while holding your breath, then begin lowering yourself back down to the floor (in the opposite sequence from the way you started) while slowly exhaling. Repeat this exercise three to five times.

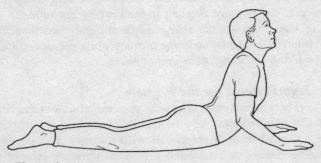

Figure 1

• **Hero Posture:** Sit on your heels and keep your back straight. Practice deep breathing until you are very relaxed. Now slowly exhale, and as you do so, separate your feet until your buttocks sink in between them and touch the floor (see **Figure 2**). Maintain this posture for about one minute, and practice it several times daily.

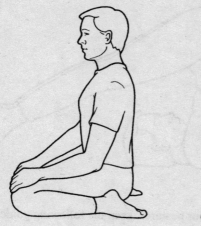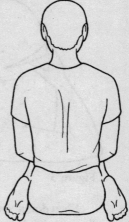

Figure 2

- **Plow Posture:** This is a slightly more difficult position and might be easier to try with the help of a friend. To do the plow, lie on your back, sliding your arms underneath your buttocks. Now raise your legs (keeping them straight) up and behind your head, until your toes are touching the floor behind you (see **Figure 3**). Your friend can help slowly guide your legs so that you don't hurt your neck or back while attaining this position. Focus on deep relaxation, and maintain slow, methodical breathing throughout the exercise. Try to maintain this position for one or two minutes.

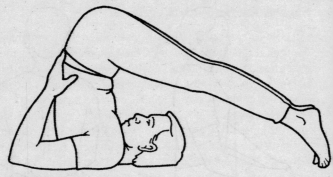

Figure 3

When doing your postures, keep the following guidelines in mind:

- Practice your sessions before meals.
- Use a well-ventilated room and make sure that you have on loose, comfortable clothing.
- Don't force your positions, and while doing them, be sure to focus on total relaxation. (Visualization techniques can be used to create mental images of tranquillity and serenity.)
- Each yoga session should not last longer than a few minutes (see under individual pose descriptions for more information).

Note: There are many more poses in yoga, and the ones we've provided are by no means a complete list. For more information, read one of the many excellent guides on yoga and its practice.

Special Exercise #3: Kegels

These exercises are usually associated with pregnancy (women do them to strengthen the pelvic and bladder muscles after childbirth). But kegels are also highly useful for helping men overcome problems such as urinary incontinence—a common side effect of prostate surgery.

To learn how to do kegels, deliberately start, then stop your urine flow—all the while being careful **NOT** to tense up any other muscles such as those in your thighs, calves, buttocks, etc. Once you can stop and start urine flow with only your bladder muscles, you've correctly learned how to do kegels, and you are now ready to practice them on a regular basis.

Try the following doctor-recommended program to get the most benefit from kegels:

- Exercise at least three times daily (morning, noon, and evening).
- During each kegel, tense up your bladder muscles for a 4-second interval, and then slowly release the tension for another 4-second interval; always be careful that you aren't tensing up nearby muscles.
- Do 10 kegels per session (for a total of 30 per day).

A Few Additional Tips

- If you are incontinent, avoid irritants such as alcohol, spices, and caffeine, all of which stimulate bladder frequency.
- Help your bladder muscles by not holding back urine for long periods of time and by making sure to visit the bathroom regularly—especially before long trips or anticipated hours away from bathroom facilities.

Reflexology

Natural healers consider *reflexology* to be one of the most beneficial forms of massage therapy for the prostate. (In mainstream medicine, direct finger massage of the prostate—via the rectum—is sometimes prescribed, and this form of massage should be performed only by a physician.)

Reflexology is the act of applying pressure to specific "zones" located on the hands and feet. These zones are described as energy pathways that link the hands and feet to the rest of the body. When the pathways become "blocked," energy flow is disrupted, leading to a state of "disharmony" and possibly illness. By applying pressure to specific zones, energy flow is stimulated and revitalized, and this is believed to promote a state of healing.

Many reports of benefit for prostate disorders have been noted via the use of reflexology, and several studies now corroborate these claims.

The Evidence

In one of the largest trials ever conducted on reflexology, 8,096 patients were treated for a number of disorders, including BPH, prostatitis, kidney and bladder problems, vertigo, respiratory infections, influenza, constipation, and diabetes. After the trial was over, lead investigator Dr. Wang Liang reported that over *90 percent of the patients* experienced clinical improvement.

Other trials have corroborated Liang's results, and additional studies are now under way to further evaluate reflexology.

Finding Your Prostate Zones

According to reflexologists, there are three main zones for your prostate. The first is located in the soft tissue below your ankle, midway between the anklebone and the Achilles tendon; the second is located directly underneath your thumb, closer to the edge of your wrist; and the third, called the "lumbar zone," is located just underneath the crease of your hand, at the midpoint of your wrist.

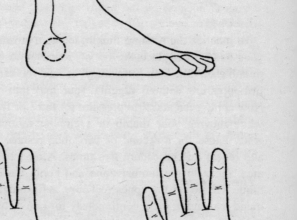

Once you've located them, begin massaging the zones by using the *rotating thumb* or *golf ball technique*.

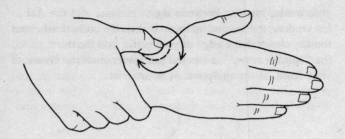

To practice the rotating thumb, locate a prostate zone on your hand, then place the tip of your thumb on it. Your thumb should be bent just enough so that you can distribute firm pressure without digging your nail into your flesh. Now apply even and firm pressure for three or four seconds while moving your thumb in a circular motion over the zone. Pause for a second or two, then resume massaging and repeat this procedure five times. After massaging this area, move to the lumbar zone and apply the same technique. (If any of the zones feel *sore,* reflexologists recommend massaging them continuously for one or two minutes until the soreness subsides.)

To massage your foot, apply the same technique, being sure to first locate the correct zone as described above. (Some reflexologists also massage the heel and the Achilles tendon, because they claim that these pathways are indirectly linked to the prostate. A pinching or squeezing motion of the fingertips is used when massaging the Achilles tendon.)

The golf ball technique is performed exactly like the rotating thumb, but instead of a finger, you use a golf ball to apply pressure. While applying firm pressure, the golf ball is moved in a small circular motion within the zone.

When to Practice Reflexology

You can do your massages at various intervals throughout the day or while you are experiencing symptoms.

Beneficial responses are said to vary considerably—with some men claiming benefit after only a few sessions, and others after a few weeks or longer. So you might want to give reflexology at least a month to assess your response.

Hydrotherapy

Whirlpools, saunas, and *baths* all come under the heading of "hydrotherapy," and all have shown a number of benefits for many disease conditions. Of these different forms of hydrotherapy, *baths* are considered the most beneficial for relieving prostatic congestion and for opening up constricted urinary passages.

Three types of baths are routinely used for the prostate: *warm baths, hot baths,* and *cold baths.*

A **warm bath** is prepared to 99°F, and it is used to relieve *acute prostatitis.* Doctors recommend sitting in the warm bath for at least half an hour.

A *hot bath* is prepared to 115°F, and it is used for *chronic prostatitis*—especially when difficult urination is present. Sit in the hot bath as long as you comfortably can (try for at least fifteen minutes), and be sure that the temperature **doesn't exceed 115°F. Caution:** Be sure to check your *water-heater temperature* before climbing in the bath to avoid scalding. You can also purchase a water thermometer and check your tub directly.

Cold baths (from 55°F to 75°F maximum) are usually used in rotation with hot baths, and these are recommended for men with *BPH* or for those recovering from *prostatitis.*

Rotation baths—in which you sit in hot and cold water in quick succession—are especially beneficial. If you don't have access to a Jacuzzi and a cold bath or pool nearby, use the following technique for doing a rotation bath at home:

Fill your bathtub about a half foot with hot water. Next to the bathtub, place a portable tub that you can comfortably sit in. Fill the portable with a half foot of cold water. Now sit in the hot tub with your legs bent toward your chest for one minute. Then quickly immerse yourself in the cold tub, adopting the same position for an equal amount of time. (This process may be repeated several times.) Try the rotation bath for several days to a week or more, until results are noted.

Note: Be sure that you move quickly from one unit of water to the other for best results. Also be careful to avoid slipping by placing a towel between the baths.

CHAPTER SEVEN

Sex and Your Prostate

Sixty-year-old Bill arranged to see his doctor because of a constant urge to urinate. After a thorough exam and some routine tests, the doctor announced that Bill was suffering from a mild case of BPH. No further medical treatment was prescribed, but the doctor did recommend something that took Bill quite by surprise: more frequent sex. According to the doctor, an increase in sexual activity could help release the buildup of semen in Bill's prostate and offset unhealthy congestion resulting from this buildup.

While Bill accepted his doctor's counsel without much difficulty, Michael—a thirty-six-year-old who was also diagnosed with BPH—took the advice given him with some reluctance. In Michael's case, the doctor suggested *less sex*—at least during the initial recovery from BPH. (It appeared that Michael's prostate problems stemmed from an overworked prostate, resulting from *too frequent* sexual activity.)

In the following sections, we'll take a closer look at sex and your prostate and then provide some doctor-recommended guidelines for helping you to decide if more—or less—is better.

Reappraising an Older Concept

The relationship between sexuality and prostate disease has had a long and controversial history. In a 1903 book published on the subject, the writer warned that sexual "over-indulgence, excessive intercourse, and masturbation" could cause lesions in the prostate. A similar account on prostate disease and sex appeared in a popular medical atlas published in 1936. According to the doctors who wrote the atlas, ". . . sexual overindulgence, masturbation . . . alcoholic intemperance, [and] a sedentary life . . . may cause the prostate to enlarge."

As the state of medicine progressed, these early-century views (*minus* the admonitions against alcohol and sedentary lifestyle) began to dissolve, and current thought held that sexuality (either with a partner or through masturbation) was not harmful. Any dangers that were related to sex were viewed in the context of disease transmission (gonorrhea, venereal disease, etc.).

Surprising as it may seem, doctors are now reevaluating the issue of sexual "overindulgence" and its possibly harmful effects on the prostate. But as mentioned earlier, there are also times when *indulgence* may help serve the prostate better, and it is here that modern medicine contrasts sharply with the older views on sex.

How Sex Affects Your Prostate

Recall from Chapter 1 the prostate's role in ejaculation and the manufacture of semen. Both of these functions are influenced by sex, and both play a key role in keeping the prostate healthy. To better understand how, consider the following illustration.

Imagine that your prostate is a production plant whose job is to keep a steady supply of semen in stock (nature designed this to ensure that there would always be enough available to keep the human race going). When the supply of semen gets too low, the prostate receives a signal from the brain to increase production. And when levels get too high, the prostate is called to release semen to avoid becoming oversaturated.

The objective is to keep a *steady* supply of semen available—not too much and not too little. However, when this delicate balance is disrupted, problems can arise. For example, if semen levels remain high for long periods of time, the ducts and other pathways that store it can become congested and inflamed. On the other hand, if levels remain too low and are not given a chance of being replenished, the prostate is forced to produce semen more quickly than it's normally capable of doing. This situation can also irritate prostate tissues and lead to a state of BPH or aggravate an existing state.

Obviously the amount of sexual activity a man has will influence his semen levels—for better or worse.

How Much Is Enough?

We can't tell you exactly how much or how little sex to have; that's a decision that must ultimately be made by you. But we can outline those sexual activities or conditions that are potentially harmful to your prostate (see below).

By identifying a circumstance that applies to you, you can then take the necessary steps to modify it. For example, if you've been sexually abstinent for many months *and* also suffer from BPH, you might want to consider having sex occasionally, or more often—because sexual abstinence is one condition that can aggravate BPH. However, if you are very sexually active and suffer from BPH, you might want to slow down or take a short rest period from sex (to allow your prostate muscles a chance to heal and for semen to be replenished).

Whatever the circumstance, remember that there are no exact rules dictating the amount of sex you should have. But with a little experimentation, you should be able to find a schedule that works best for you.

SEXUAL CONDITIONS OR ACTIVITIES THAT CAN AGGRAVATE YOUR PROSTATE

- **Total sexual abstinence.** No release of semen for extended or unusually long periods of time is potentially harmful to the prostate.
- **Too much sexual activity.** This can be determined by the amount of time it takes for your semen levels to restore themselves *between* periods of sex. In a younger man of twenty, semen levels can be replenished in a few hours, whereas in an older man of sixty, two or three days might be the norm. Not waiting for the levels to replenish before having sex again is considered overdoing it if you have prostate disease.
- **Prolonged intercourse or delayed orgasm.** They might be popular in the movies and in the media, but long, drawn-out lovemaking sessions *can* bother your prostate—especially if you are at risk for or already suffer from BPH. This occurs because long periods of sexual arousal cause high semen levels in the prostate, and this leads to congestion and further inflammation. By the same token, continued arousal without ejaculation may

also lead to a prolonged and unhealthy state of seminal congestion.

- **A sudden increase in sexual activity.** In healthy men semen levels manufactured by the prostate typically adjust to the normal routine of sexual activity; however, any deviation in this activity (for example, going from two sessions of sex weekly to one per day) can affect the prostate adversely.

- **Ejaculatory failure or impotence.** Men who can perform sexually but are unable to ejaculate are at higher risk for prostate disease. Similarly, men who suffer from impotence but experience long periods of arousal while attempting erection are also at risk. In both cases, ejaculation should be attempted. (For men with ejaculatory failure or impotence, orgasm can sometimes be achieved through masturbation—especially when psychological factors are involved.)

An Exception to the Rule

In cases of chronic BPH and prostatitis, some doctors recommend short periods of abstinence (or "vacations") from sex that last for a few days to a week or more, just to allow the gland a chance to recuperate.

If improvements are noted, the abstinence period ends and the guidelines discussed in this chapter may be followed accordingly. However, if no improvements are noted, the abstinence period can be discontinued.

A Few Other Considerations

Besides the issue of *how much* sex is healthy for your prostate, the potential dangers caused by *disease transmission* are also important factors to keep in mind.

Any virus or bacterium that you're exposed to during sex can affect your prostate. For example, unprotected anal intercourse can introduce dangerous bacteria into the penis through the urinary tract and then into the prostate; penile-vaginal intercourse can also expose a man to urinary-tract infections with eventual prostate involvement.

One of the oldest and most effective methods for protecting yourself from disease transmission is to wear a condom. But although condoms can protect you against bacteria, ultrathin condoms (made from sheepskin or lambskin) may not prevent infection against the extremely small AIDS virus. For this reason, health experts recommend using the thicker latex condoms with added spermicide.

The Medical Benefits of Monogamy

Having sex with one partner in a long-term relationship may not be suitable for everyone. But it is true that *knowing* your partner for a long time can help tip the scales *against* your contracting a sexually transmitted disease. In this regard, you're more likely to know if your wife or steady lover suffers from an STD or a UTI than you would a total stranger.

CHAPTER EIGHT

What You Need to Know About Prostate Cancer

Two hundred thousand men are diagnosed with prostate cancer every year in the United States, and 40,000 die from it. In fact, this disease is the most common form of cancer among men and ranks second—only to lung cancer—as a killer of men aged fifty and older.

Prostate cancer may be far more common than is generally realized. According to experts, about *one third* of men over the age of fifty and *one half* of men over the age of eighty have some evidence of the disease. But fortunately most of these men will lead completely normal lives and never experience any symptoms, because undetected prostate cancer is often very slow growing.

For those men who have been diagnosed and who are symptomatic, prostate cancer can usually be cured—if the disease is caught early enough. And treatments are also available that can extend life span in more advanced cases of cancer.

What Causes It?

Dietary fat, high cholesterol, environmental toxins such as pesticides, and genetic factors are all believed to play a role in causing prostate cancer. The hormone testosterone may also be a causative factor; besides promoting the overgrowth of prostate tissues as seen in BPH, testosterone also fuels cancer once the disease has started.

Symptoms of Prostate Cancer

Frequency, nighttime urination, difficulty in starting urination, incomplete emptying, and virtually any of the symptoms that apply to BPH or prostatitis can also signal prostate cancer. In addition, *hematuria* (i.e., blood in the urine) is a very important symptom. Not infrequently, hematuria is invisible to the naked eye and requires laboratory testing to determine its presence.

The above symptoms should always be investigated promptly.

How It Is Diagnosed

Nearly half of all prostate cancers are diagnosed early enough to be successfully treated. The key to early diagnosis is having an annual physical that includes rectal examination, PSA testing, and urinalysis.

Interestingly, prostate cancer is probably found as much via rectal examination as by any other diagnostic technique. The rectal exam—technically called *anal-digital examination*—allows the doctor to feel (or palpate) the prostate for any irregularities. Most doctors recommend rectal examination to all men over the age of forty.

Physicians also routinely use the *prostate-specific antigen* (or PSA test) to screen for cancer. PSA testing checks for levels of a particular protein that, if elevated, indicates the possibility of cancer but *does not prove* its presence. For middle-aged men, a "normal" PSA reading is considered to be 4.0 or under; as men reach the seventh decade of life, PSA readings may climb—with normal values hovering around 6.5.

While the PSA is helpful in diagnosing cancer, it is not an entirely accurate test. In fact, the following conditions may cause PSA readings to fluctuate, masking the true presence of cancer or suggesting cancer when there is none:

- A prostate that weighs more than average may cause a higher-than-average PSA reading.
- A smaller-than-normal prostate can generate "normal" PSA readings that in actuality might be relatively *high* for a smaller prostate.
- Certain medications such as Proscar and natural substances such as saw palmetto can cause PSA levels to go down.
- Infections can cause PSA levels to rise.
- Rectal finger examination may cause small increases in PSA levels.

Doctors are now refining the PSA with other procedures to help improve diagnostic accuracy. For example, ultrasound is one test that can help to determine true prostate size—relative to a patient's PSA readings. With ultrasound, a more accurate interpretation of PSA results can then be made.

Other Diagnostic Tests

If cancer is suspected, a biopsy is usually performed, as well as additional blood tests to help determine whether cancer has spread beyond the prostate. Once cancer has been firmly diagnosed, secondary tests might include an *MRI* (magnetic resonance imaging) and ultrasound. These tests scan bodily organs for the presence of distant cancer cells or tumors.

MRI and ultrasound are used less for diagnostic purposes than to *stage* the cancer—an important first step in helping the physician decide on the best course of treatment (see the sidebar for a description of prostate cancer stages and their average cure rates).

Surgical Treatment for Prostate Cancer

The mainstay of treatment for localized prostate cancer is surgery, with or without radiation. But for men who are in their seventies or older, surgery may not be the only treatment option, because prostate cancers tend to grow very slowly in older men and don't always pose a threat. In these cases, simply monitoring the cancer (''watchful waiting'') is considered a possible alternative to surgery.

Though it is still controversial, there *is* compelling evidence that watchful waiting may yield about the same survival advantages as surgery for some patients. Of course, the decision to opt for watchful waiting is one that should be made only after careful consideration of a patient's age, diagnosis, type of tumor, quality of life, etc.

In younger men watchful waiting is not usually an option, because prostate cancers are typically more aggressive. However, exceptions are sometimes made for younger patients who are in poor or frail health.

For patients with advanced cancers that have spread beyond the prostate, surgery is usually not performed regardless of age, because such an operation would have little curative value; in addition, the side effects would outweigh any potential gains.

In these cases, other treatments (including radiation and/or hormone therapies) are sometimes used.

FIVE-YEAR PROSTATE CANCER SURVIVAL RATES ACCORDING TO STAGE

Stage of Cancer	Description	Five-Year Survival Rate
Stage A1	The tumor is localized to an area in size less than 5% of the prostate	Almost all men will survive this stage, with or without treatment
Stage A2	This tumor is more aggressive than A1 and occupies a larger area of the prostate	60%
Stage B1	The tumor is limited to one lobe of the prostate	75%
Stage B2	The tumor penetrates more than one lobe	60%

Stage C1	The tumor has spread beyond the prostate	50%–55%
Stage C2	The tumor has spread beyond the prostate and also involves nearby tissues	40%–45%
Stage D1	Cancer cells are found in the lymph nodes	40%
Stage D2	In addition to the lymph nodes, cancer has spread to distant organs	35%

The *radical retropubic prostatectomy* (or RRP) is one of the most common types of surgery for prostate cancer. It involves cutting into the lower abdomen and then completely excising (or removing) the prostate, along with the seminal vesicles (the tubes that carry sperm through the prostate) and the adjacent lymph nodes. This operation is a complex one and often causes major side effects.

Another type of surgery is known as the *radical perineal prostatectomy* (or RPP), and it's considered safer because the prostate is removed through an incision in the *perineum* (the area of tissue between the scrotum and the anus). With the RPP, major abdominal surgery—with its many complications—can be avoided.

Both types of prostate surgery offer certain advantages and disadvantages, as we will now see.

RRP versus RPP: Pros and Cons

Infections, bleeding, pain, incontinence, impotence, and a long convalescence have all been common side effects of the radical retropubic prostatectomy. But in spite of these significant problems, many surgeons feel this is the best treatment approach for prostate cancer. They explain that RRP allows for easier removal of the prostate without damaging those nerves involved in erection. (However, not all patients retain their ability to have an erection, even after nerve-sparing surgery has been performed.)

RRP also allows for lymph nodes to be removed from the abdomen, and these nodes can then be quickly "sampled" to see if cancer has spread beyond the prostate. If the samples are negative, the prostate is removed. But if they are positive and there is evidence of cancer spread, most surgeons will not remove the prostate; as explained earlier, such an operation would have little curative value.

Other surgeons claim that the radical perineal prostatectomy is better because it results in fewer complications and a much quicker recovery.

One problem with the RPP is that lymph nodes can't be removed via the perineum. However, a procedure known as *laparoscopic lymphadenectomy* (or *LL*) allows for lymph nodes to be removed *before* patients undergo RPP. Then, after the lymph nodes are examined, a decision for or against surgery can be made.

An additional problem with RPP is a greater likelihood of damage to prostatic nerves—and resultant impotence. But impotence appears less likely to occur when RPPs are performed by experienced surgeons.

At this time the jury is still out on which surgery is better for prostate cancer. But regardless of the type of surgery performed, steps can be taken to improve the outcome—and this has to do with one's choice of surgeon.

According to Dr. Patrick Walsh, who pioneered nerve-sparing prostate surgery, one important indicator of a surgeon's skill and efficiency is the amount of surgery he or she performs yearly (with 150 or more cases being considered ideal). Another indicator is the surgeon's track record. For example, what percentage of patients recover full use of their sexuality? How many remain cancer free five years or longer? How many are incontinent, and how many require a long convalescence after surgery? Answering these questions and developing a profile on the doctor that you choose might very well tip the odds in favor of a more successful treatment experience.

Radiation Therapy

When cancer isn't curable by surgery, or when there's evidence of malignancy outside of the prostate, radiation can be used as an optional therapy. In some cases of localized cancer, doctors recommend radiation in addition to surgery, to ensure that all malignant cells have been destroyed.

Two types of radiation therapy are used for prostate cancer. *External beam radiation* is administered to a small area of the abdomen and used to reach a specific target inside of or directly around the prostate. *Interstitial radiation* involves the implanting of small radioactive seeds directly into the prostate. This procedure is done via surgical incision.

Both therapies have potentially serious drawbacks comparable to the side effects of surgery.

External radiation can cause severe incontinence, urgency, painful urination, impotence, rectal pain, spasms, and severe diarrhea. The side effects from radioactive implants are not as pronounced, but improperly placed seeds can cause incomplete destruction of malignant cells. There can also be damage to the lining of the rectum that causes urine to pass through the bowel and feces to pass through the urinary tract. These side effects appear less likely to occur, however, when interstitial radiation is correctly performed by a highly qualified surgeon.

Hormone Therapies

Cancers that are not curable by either surgery or radiation often respond very well to hormone therapies; these are occasionally effective in slowing or even stopping the growth of cancer for long periods of time. The premise behind hormone therapy is to block the production of testosterone, which acts as a stimulant of prostate cancer growth.

For many decades *estrogen* has been the hormone of choice for prostate cancer because of its antitestosterone effects. In addition *orchiectomy*—which is surgical removal of the testicles, the major source of testosterone in men—had also been commonly performed. But today estrogen therapy and surgical castration are used far less often, and in their place *nonestrogen* drugs are being used. These are considered a major improvement, because the side effects associated with estrogen (which include enlargement of the breasts, hair loss, weight gain, hot flashes, impotence, loss of sexual desire, heart irregularities, blood clots, and stroke) are considerably less.

There are two classes of nonestrogen drugs, and they are called *LHRH agonists* and *antiandrogens*. The two types can be used together to effectively stop hormone production in different parts of the body. For example, LHRH agonists prevent the testicles from making testosterone, while antiandrogens block testosterone production in the adrenal glands. With this dual approach, a nearly complete shutdown of testosterone can be achieved.

Luprolide, goserelin, flutamide, and *bicalutamide* are a few of the LHRH agonists and antiandrogens now on the market.

Nonestrogen Drugs: Pros and Cons

One advantage of taking LHRHs and antiandrogens is that they cause fewer estrogenesque effects such as breast enlargement and hair loss. However, problems can still occur.

The treatments can result in a temporary *rise* in testosterone levels, adrenal difficulties, blood-clotting problems, high blood pressure, malaise, and weight gain. Perhaps more common, these drugs tend to have a negative effect on mood, causing anxiety and depression in some patients.

A change of drug or a lower dosage can reduce side effects. For this reason, it's important that patients be monitored continuously while undergoing therapy.

Experimental Treatments Under Investigation

In spite of much progress, surgery, radiation, and hormone therapies have not proved totally effective for prostate cancer. In addition, questions about side effects and the quality of life proffered by these treatments are now being debated in many circles. With such critical issues in mind, researchers are now experimenting with newer and more innovative ways to treat and hopefully cure prostate cancer.

Following are two such therapies now under evaluation by the National Cancer Institute (NCI):

Hyperthermia is the use of heat to kill cancer cells. Hyperthermia was once considered an "alternative" therapy, but it's now receiving more acceptance in mainstream medicine.

Various techniques are used in hyperthermia. One involves the insertion of plastic or fiber-optic cylinders into the prostate; bursts of microwave or ultrasound energy are then delivered through the cylinders and directly into the tumors.

Another technique uses magnetic rods or sapphire probes that deliver laser-generated heat to tumors.

Whole body hyperthermia employs special probes or water-filled blankets to raise total body temperature. This procedure is considered beneficial when cancer cells have spread to distant sites throughout the body.

The best results against prostate cancer thus far have been achieved when hyperthermia is combined with radiation. One of the advantages of this dual approach is that smaller-than-normal amounts of radiation can be used to shrink tumors.

If hyperthermia and radiation cause enough reduction in tumor size, patients may become candidates for curative surgery.

Cryosurgery works in the _opposite_ way to hyperthermia. Instead of being destroyed by heating, cancer cells are immobilized by _freezing_.

Cryosurgery is performed by inserting special probes through the perineum and into the prostate. (These probes must be placed in precise locations to be effective.) Once in place, the probes are filled with extremely cold *liquid nitrogen,* and this destroys cancer cells.

Cryosurgery is considered a safe and feasible option for men who are unable to undergo radical surgery. But while cryosurgery is less invasive, side effects can still be *similar* to those of surgery. For example, incontinence, difficulty in urinating, perineal pain, and other disabling problems have all resulted from cryosurgery. In addition, damage to the urethra can cause the passing of urine through the bowel (in much the same way that radiation damage causes this effect). Worse, impotence is an *expected side effect* of cryosurgery.

At this point, there is still debate as to cryosurgery's real benefits. Adding to the debate are several studies that show a "significant complication rate"—especially among patients who have already undergone radiation treatments.

In the next chapter, we're going to look at complementary cancer therapies that are considered less toxic than some of the treatments discussed so far.

CHAPTER NINE

Complementary Approaches for Treating Prostate Cancer

In a recent Gallup poll, one third of Americans diagnosed with cancer said they had used complementary treatment approaches during the course of their illness.[1] When asked why, some people explained that they were disillusioned with the standard therapies; for example, the side effects of toxic chemotherapy and radiation, and the traumatic aftereffects of major cancer surgery were among the most common reasons cited. Others felt that they had benefited from conventional treatments but wanted to improve their overall health and recovery with natural medicines and strategies.

What a Complementary Program Can Do for You

If you have prostate cancer, a complementary program can help you achieve the following goals:

[1] In the context of cancer therapies, the term *complementary* generally refers to natural as well as other body-friendly treatments that are used to help bolster immunity and the body's healing forces.

- improve your cancer-fighting immunity
- inhibit tumor growth in some cases
- improve the outcome of conventional treatments
- overcome treatment-related side effects
- maximize your recovery from cancer

The complementary approaches discussed in this chapter include *dietary interventions, nutrient therapies, immunological programs, herbal medicine* and *mind-body techniques*. In addition, the controversial *antineoplaston* therapy of Dr. Stanislaw Burzynski and the much-publicized cancer drug *hydrazine sulfate* will be discussed.

All of these programs can be used to strengthen your cancer-fighting immunity and to help you cope with the side effects of conventional treatments you may be receiving.

How Safe Are Complementary Medicines?

The strategies discussed in this chapter are generally safe, but there are a few exceptions. For example, you might not be a good candidate for a therapeutic diet if you are experiencing progressive weight loss or are undernourished as the result of surgery or illness. You might also experience problems using a complementary drug like hydrazine sulfate if you are receiving medications for depression. (These and other potential problems and side effects from treatments will be listed as necessary.)

The decision to embark on a complementary program is one that you should make only after speaking with your doctor. If your doctor is not open to the idea, consult with a clinician who is and who can provide you with close support. This way your progress can be monitored, and any problems that you may run into, averted.

How to Use This Chapter

The information in this chapter can be used to help both you and your doctor plan a complementary program for cancer. For example, you can begin following a therapeutic diet or a vitamin regimen as described in the sections "**Dietary Interventions**," and "**Vitamin C and Other Nutrient Therapies**"; other treatment suggestions are described under their respective subheadings, and these can be followed accordingly.

You can also use the following information to help you evaluate clinics or hospitals that specialize in diet, vitamins, or other complementary treatments. (See Appendix 2 for a full listing of clinics, hospitals, and physicians that offer the therapies discussed in this chapter.)

Dietary Interventions

The role of diet in _cancer prevention_ is now considered a fairly well established fact. But can special diets play a role in _cancer treatment_? There's been much debate over this question, but many clinicians are convinced that diet does have an enormous impact on the growth of cancer. These clinicians say that lowering fat intake, eliminating most animal foods, eating fruits and vegetables rich in specific nutrients, and lowering (or avoiding) sodium can inhibit cancer growth.

THE EVIDENCE

Several compelling studies are supporting the benefits of special diets in cancer treatment.

In a 1990 study, researchers from the Austrian Department of General Surgery found that terminally ill colon cancer patients who were treated with a vegetarian low-salt diet survived longer than patients not receiving such a diet.

Diet therapy also helped to reverse or control weight loss, prevented dangerous complications associated with cancer, and eliminated the need for pain medication in most of the patients.

Perhaps two of the most intriguing studies ever conducted on diet and cancer involved the Japanese dietary program known as *macrobiotics.*

In the first study, four out of six patients with "medically incurable" cancers experienced "significant or total remissions" from macrobiotic treatment. One of the patients who was diagnosed with incurable pancreatic cancer was "alive and well" nine years after diagnosis, and another with malignant melanoma remained in complete remission for nine years.

In the second study, conducted by the Tulane School of Public Health, twenty-four advanced cancer patients were compared with a control group of patients who didn't receive macrobiotics. According to the Tulane report, **the mean survival rate for the macrobiotic patients was *triple* that of their counterparts.**

There have also been individual reports of prostate cancer patients benefiting from diet therapies. For example, one patient diagnosed with "adenocarcinoma of the prostate" experienced a "complete remission" after following the diet therapy (see page 112) of the late Dr. Max Gerson.

In a similar case, a man who had a positive biopsy for prostate cancer in 1976 was found to be clear of cancer one year after undergoing similar treatment; as of 1991, follow-up testing showed no sign of cancer.

WHAT ARE THERAPEUTIC DIETS LIKE?

While there are variations, most anticancer diets have several points of similarity. The following recommendations and suggestions are typical of most of these diets:

Prohibited Foods

- Refined foods
- Fatty, fried, or smoked foods
- Iron-rich foods
- Dairy products (except the limited amounts that may be prescribed)
- Canned soups
- Sprayed, canned, or frozen vegetables
- Vegetables high in sodium
- Sodium, table salt, salty foods, salt substitutes
- Roasted, salted nuts
- Fats and saturated oils
- Bleached, enriched flours
- Sugar, spices
- Custards, pastries, puddings, ice creams
- Drinking water (so that juices are drunk exclusively)
- Alcohol, cocoa, coffee

Recommended Foods

- Baked or boiled potatoes, whole-grain breads (five-grain, etc.), oatmeal, barley, millet, brown rice, wild rice
- Fresh fruits and juices, freshly cooked vegetables, raw vegetables, homemade vegetable soups, fresh salads
- Soybeans, soy products (miso, shoyu, tempeh, tofu)
- Fresh raw nuts
- Olive, canola, and sesame oils
- Chives, garlic, onion, parsley, sage, thyme, sea salt, kelp, sesame salt, etc.
- Nut milks (made from almonds or cashews); seed milks (made from sunflower seeds, sesame seeds, etc.)

Optional

- Fish (freshwater and sea fish, broiled, baked, or poached)
- Chicken (prohibited in some therapeutic diets because of the belief that cancer-causing bacteria may infect poultry)
- Sea vegetables (brown kelp or kombu, wakame, nori, dulse), shiitake mushrooms

Sample Diets

Livingston Clinic Daily Menu

Breakfast

8-oz. glass carrot juice containing ¼ avocado
Basic millet with nut milk
Whole-grain toast, if desired
Violet leaf tea

Lunch

Grated carrot with mixed vegetable salad and horseradish
  dressing
Black bean soup
Curried vegetables
Vegetable snack: choice of squash, okra, zucchini, celery,
  carrots, turnip, or parsnip (raw)
Whole-grain bread and butter
Strawberry leaf tea

Dinner

Mixed vegetable salad
Cream of mushroom soup
Spaghetti squash
Whole-grain bread and butter
Peppermint leaf tea

Gerson Therapy Daily Menu

Breakfast

1 glass juice
Large portion of oatmeal
Bread (dark rye, toasted or plain) with honey or stewed
  fruit

Lunch

Salad (raw food)
Pot cheese and buttermilk (as prescribed)

1 glass warm soup, 1 glass juice
Large baked potato
Vegetables, cooked
Dessert: raw or stewed fruit

Dinner
Salad
Pot cheese and buttermilk (as prescribed)
1 glass warm soup
1 glass juice
Large baked potato
2 vegetables, cooked
Dessert: raw or stewed fruit

ADDITIONAL HOURLY JUICE SCHEDULE*

Time	Juice	
8:00 A.M.	Orange	Breakfast
9:00	Green†	
10:00	Apple-carrot	
11:00	Liver	
12:00 P.M.	Green	
1:00	Apple-carrot	Lunch
2:00	Green	
3:00	Liver	
4:00	Liver	
5:00	Apple-carrot	
5:30	Apple-carrot	
6:00	Green	
7:00	Apple-carrot	Dinner

* Juices are freshly prepared in a high-quality juicer using only organic, pesticide-free fruits, vegetables, and fresh organic calf's liver
† Green juice consists of lettuce, red cabbage, escarole, green pepper, and watercress.

Macrobiotic Daily Menu

Breakfast
Miso soup
Soft brown rice with kombu
    and shiitake mushrooms
Bancha tea

Lunch
Udon and broth
Steamed brussels sprouts
Garden salad
Bancha tea

Dinner
Pressure-cooked brown rice
Soybean casserole
Steamed mustard greens
Hijiki with onion
Cooked peaches
Bancha tea

Between-Meal Snacks
Mochi (a sweet rice served in cakes or squares)
Noodles
Popcorn
Puffed whole cereal grains
Rice balls, cakes
Seeds
Vegetable sushi

Vitamin C and Other Nutrient Therapies

Vitamin C: Perhaps no other vitamin has received as much attention for its role in cancer treatment as vitamin C. Indeed, many nutritionally oriented physicians believe that vitamin C is one of the single most important nutrients that should be administered to all cancer patients—regardless of what other therapy they may be receiving.

The use of vitamin C in cancer treatment stems from research conducted by the late Nobel laureate Linus Pauling and his colleague Dr. Ewan Cameron. In one of their first collaborations, Pauling and Cameron treated a small number of advanced cancer patients at the Vale of Leven Hospital in Scotland. The patients were given 10 grams (10,000 mg) of vitamin C daily, and this dosage was said to have achieved striking results for some of the patients.

In a second carefully controlled trial, Pauling and Cameron treated 100 terminally ill cancer patients and then compared them with 1,000 patients who didn't receive vitamin C. After a five-year follow-up, Cameron and Pauling announced that the vitamin-treated patients lived significantly longer than the control group—in some cases they had *double* the life span of the control group.

Recommended dosage for prostate cancer is 1 to 10 or more grams daily in the form of *ascorbic acid* tablets or capsules. The salt version of vitamin C (*sodium ascorbate*) is **NOT** recommended for long-term use.

Vitamin C should be taken in gradually increasing dosages until *bowel tolerance* (symptoms of gas, diarrhea, bloating, etc.) occurs. After bowel tolerance is reached, the dosage should be scaled back until symptoms subside; this is considered the optimal therapeutic dose of vitamin C.

Side effects other than those occurring from bowel tolerance are not generally considered a problem with vitamin C therapy.

(See Appendix 1 for more information on vitamin C and bowel tolerance.)

A number of practitioners prescribe vitamin C along with other nutrients as part of a comprehensive program to treat prostate cancer. These substances are administered in pill or tablet form and in some cases intravenously.

Among the nutrients most often prescribed are the following:

Vitamin A: Hundreds of animal studies conducted over the last seventy years have shown this vitamin's cancer-inhibiting effects. Recent human trials also show strong protective effects from vitamin A and in some cases treatment benefits.

Recommended dosage of vitamin A in cancer treatment is generally 25,000 IU to 50,000 IU daily. Because of the potential for vitamin A toxicity, **beta-carotene** should be taken instead (beta-carotene is converted by the body into vitamin A *as needed*).

Comparable dosages are between 15,000 IU and 30,000 IU (10–20 mg) of beta-carotene daily.

Selenium: This mineral has shown potent antitumor effects in animals and strong protective/inhibitory effects in humans.

Recommended Dosage: Selenium can be toxic in doses higher than 300 micrograms daily, but some physicians prescribe higher amounts for cancer patients. Other doctors also administer selenium in fatty solutions known as *lipids;* given this way, selenium is relatively nontoxic and can be given in higher-than-normal amounts.

Coenzyme Q10: A nutrient/enzyme with many favorable effects, coenzyme Q10 (CQ10) can improve cancer-fighting immunity and also protect the heart from the toxic effects of chemotherapy.

Recommended dosage is from 30 milligrams to 150 milligrams daily. Although CQ10 is relatively nontoxic, side effects can occur from what's known as the *rebound effect;* this occurs when CQ10 is suddenly discontinued and people experience a worsening of their symptoms.

To avoid the rebound effect, don't discontinue taking CQ10 until you've reduced the dosage gradually.

Germanium: Prescribed more commonly in Japan, this mineral improves immunity and has been shown to inhibit tumor growth. Organic forms are considered safer than nonorganic forms such as germanium oxide (the latter can cause kidney damage). Because of potentially serious side effects, germanium should be taken only under the supervision of a practitioner.

Shark cartilage: Since the highly popular book *Sharks Don't Get Cancer* was published a few years ago, shark cartilage has received much publicity. Though not strictly a *nutrient,* shark cartilage does appear to harness the body's natural resources the way that nutrients do.

In several studies, shark cartilage has been found to choke off the blood vessels that feed tumors. Small studies also suggest that shark cartilage can inhibit tumor growth in humans. Therapeutic doses of this substance are in the range of 30 grams or more daily; however, smaller amounts may be beneficial to some cancer patients.

Recommended dosage for cancer patients is from several to 30 grams of shark cartilage daily. The prescribed dosages are considered safe and nontoxic. Consult with a naturopath or other clinician for additional advice.

Immunity-Boosting Cancer Programs

A number of physicians use nontoxic vaccines in an effort to help the body fight cancer. These vaccines, unlike toxic chemotherapy, work with and not against the body's natural defenses.

One proponent of nontoxic vaccines in cancer treatment is Dr. Burton Waisbren. Dr. Waisbren developed his program after conducting a carefully controlled research study involving 139 cancer patients.

In the study, vaccine-treated cancer patients were followed for a period of eleven years. At study's end, survival rates were found to be statistically better compared with similar patients who received only standard treatments. Other studies have corroborated these results.

Specifically, the Waisbren program (which can be used in conjunction with other immune-friendly therapies such as diet and nutrition) consists of the following four vaccines:

- *Mixed bacterial vaccine* (made from several strains of bacteria that cause immune-system responses in people)
- **Transfer factor** (made from special immune-system cells taken from healthy donors)
- *BCG* (a vaccine used for TB that has now been approved by the NCI for the treatment of bladder cancer; a genetically engineered form of BCG has also shown positive effects against melanoma and leukemia and may be indicated as an appropriate adjuvant therapy for prostate cancer)
- *Lymphoblastoid lymphocytes* (made from healthy immune systems actively fighting infections)

Dr. Waisbren believes that all cancer patients can benefit from immunity-enhancing programs such as his. He emphasizes that the addition of nontoxic immunotherapy programs can increase the odds in favor of recovery from cancer or improve relapse-free survival. You can't purchase adjuvant vaccines yourself, so you'll need to consult with a physician who does.

Herbal Medicine

Much interest is now being generated over the use of herbs in cancer treatment. In fact, studies are showing that herbs possess a wide range of anticancer activity. (Refer to Chapter 3 for information on how to buy and prepare herbs.)

You can experiment with medicinal herbs yourself—provided that dosage suggestions are followed carefully. However, you should **NOT** take **pokeweed** (described below) unless you are under the care of a physician or practitioner who specializes in herbal medicine. See the resource listings in Appendix 2 for information on finding a qualified herbalist.

The following are considered among the most beneficial herbs for cancer:

Buckthorn: Contains the chemical *aloe emodin,* which shows effects against animal leukemias and cancer.
Recommended Dosage and Usage: As a *tea,* 1 to 3 cups daily. In *capsule* form, 1 to 3 daily.
Side Effects: Use of the fresh plant may cause cramps and vomiting. Always start with smaller amounts of buckthorn, then build up the dosage gradually while watching for any possible side effects.

Burdock: Has been found to contain a substance that prevents cells from mutating and becoming abnormal. The herb also shows effects against HIV and other viruses.
Recommended Dosage and Usage: Burdock may be taken in *capsule* form (a maximum of 3 per day); as an *extract* (10–25 drops daily, mixed with juice); or as a *tea* (3

bags per cup of boiling water). Smaller doses should be used at first, and these can be increased gradually.

Side Effects: High doses of burdock can provoke toxic conditions in the body. Also, burdock is *rich in iron;* those concerned with overdoing iron intake should take caution.

Echinacea: Bolsters immune-system functions involved in the cancer process. For example, echinacea improves T-cell function (T cells influence the activity of cancer-fighting cells) and also stimulates the production of interferon (a crucial blood protein that fights cancer). The leaves and roots are used to prepare echinacea.

Recommended Dosage and Usage: Echinacea may be taken in *capsule* form (1–3 daily); as an *extract* (15–30 drops up to 4 times daily); as a *tincture* (1–3 teaspoons daily); or as a *decoction* (1–3 cups daily).

Side Effects: Echinacea is considered a very safe herb.

Licorice Root: May play a very useful role in cancer treatment, according to recent studies conducted by the National Cancer Institute's Experimental Food Program.

Recommended Dosage and Usage: Licorice root can be taken in *capsule* form (1–3 times daily); as a *decoction* (1–2 cups daily); as a *tincture* (1/2–1 teaspoon, 1–3 times daily); or as an *extract* (1/2–1 teaspoon, 1–3 times daily). Because of this herb's potency, you should use it only in the recommended doses.

Side Effects: Adverse effects include headache, swelling, and fatigue. If you suffer from high blood pressure or glaucoma, you should take licorice root only under expert supervision.

Pau D'arco: Has shown a broad spectrum of benefits against cancer and other diseases. One of the prime ingredients of pau d'arco is a chemical known as _lapachol,_ which belongs to a family of substances with anticancer activity.

Recommended Dosage and Usage: Pau d'arco can be taken in _capsule_ form (1–3 daily); as an _extract_ (20–40 drops mixed with juice 3 times daily); as a _decoction_ (1–3 cups daily); or as a _tincture_ (1–3 teaspoons daily). Use only the form of pau d'arco containing lapachol. The _Tabebuia impetiginosa_ and _Tabebuia heptaphylla_ trees are believed to contain the most concentrated levels of this substance.

Side Effects: Large amounts of lapachol can cause blood-clotting problems, adverse effects on blood sugar, and other potentially serious side effects in some people. Several experts point out, however, that the doses of lapachol that cause these problems are far greater than those normally recommended.

Pokeweed: Antibodylike chemicals from pokeweed selectively target certain cancer cells. Pokeweed also stimulates the body's production of T and B cells and interleukins—key immune-system proteins that fight cancer. Another important property of pokeweed is its ability to regulate cell division; a lack of regulation is what distinguishes cancer cells from normally dividing cells.

Caution: Only the **_dried root_** is used to prepare pokeweed since the **berries and fresh leaves are POISONOUS. DO NOT** use pokeweed unless directed by your health practitioner.

Recommended Dosage and Usage: Pokeweed is so potent that only 1 to 3 teaspoonfuls are given as a decoction; in extract form, some herbalists administer 3 to 10 drops.

Pokeweed root can be purchased through some herbal distribution houses, but because of toxicity, never experiment with this plant unless you are under the close supervision of a licensed herbalist or other health professional.

Side Effects: Adverse effects include stomach cramps, diarrhea, nausea, and vomiting.

Red Clover: Has long been known for its antitumor properties. Recent research is now finding that red clover contains antioxidant and cancer-inhibiting chemicals that may be effective against certain forms of cancer.

Recommended Dosage and Usage: Red clover can be taken as an *infusion* (1–3 cups daily); as a *tincture* (1/2–1 1/2 teaspoons, 3 times daily); or in *capsule* form (check labeling recommendations).

Side Effects: Generally considered a safe herb.

Herbal Combinations for Cancer

Research shows that different herbs exhibit different kinds of activity against cancer. For this reason, experts recommend using herbal combinations to derive maximum benefit.

One of the oldest and best-known herbal combinations is *Essiac tea.* The tea can be purchased in health food stores (it is quite expensive), or you can prepare it yourself. The following is one popular recipe for making Essiac tea:

Take 6 1/2 ounces of cut burdock root, 16 ounces of sheep sorrel herb (powder), 1 ounce of turkey rhubarb root (powder), and 4 ounces of slippery elm bark (powder). Mix them thoroughly, then bring 2 gallons of distilled water to a brisk boil in a stainless steel kettle and boil for about 30 minutes. Stir 8 ounces of the herbs into the boiling water for 10 minutes, and then allow to cool for several hours. (You can use the remaining dry herbs to make additional tea later.)

Once it has cooled, stir the formula thoroughly with a wooden spoon and let it settle for another few hours.

Return the kettle to the stove, bring it to another quick boil, then pour the tea through a stainless steel strainer into a second kettle. Clean the first kettle thoroughly, then strain the contents from kettle two into kettle one. Bottle the tea immediately into dark amber glass bottles (available from some pharmacies) and seal it while still hot. Store in the refrigerator.

To use Essiac, heat 2 ounces (approximately 4 table-spoons) of distilled water, then mix this with 2 ounces of the tea taken directly from your refrigerator. (Essiac should be taken at bedtime on an empty stomach at least 2 hours after eating.) Shake well each time before pouring.

Herbal combinations with anticancer activity can also be purchased in capsule form, and many health and retail stores carry these products.

One product called **Red Clover Combination** is sold by the company Nature's Way. It contains buckthorn, burdock, licorice root, barberry, echinacea, and other ingredients.

A similar product (also called **Red Clover Combination**) is distributed by Nature's Resource. It contains buckthorn, burdock, pau d'arco, and sheep sorrel (the ingredient found in Essiac tea).

Antineoplastons

Developed by a Polish émigré named Stanislaw Burzynski, antineoplastons are medicines that help the body's own defenses overcome cancer. Antineoplastons (originally made from the urine of cancer patients) have been found to suppress the activity of cancer-causing genes while also regulating cell growth.

In one study involving twelve prostate cancer patients, two experienced "complete remissions," three had "partial remissions," and seven had "objective stabilization" after undergoing antineoplaston therapy. Clinical improvement was accompanied by a drop in cancer markers and an improvement in bone scans.

PAST DISPUTES BETWEEN DR. BURZYNSKI AND THE FDA

Even though Dr. Burzynski has published hundreds of peer-reviewed articles and has carefully followed the protocols of scientific investigation, there have been past disagreements over his use of antineoplastons.

One of the chief problems facing the Texas doctor has been his distribution of antineoplastons to patients outside the state; because these medicines are not yet fully approved by the FDA, their transport across state lines has resulted in court actions involving breaches of mail fraud laws. However, *all* of these allegations have so far ended in acquittals—the last occurring in a highly publicized May 1997 trial.

Despite the disputes between Dr. Burzynski and the FDA, a large and loyal following of cancer patients and supporters continue to protest any legal or other challenges facing the physician. In addition, the National Cancer Institute has also shown an interest in antineoplastons. And at this time a number of clinical trials are being conducted to determine the exact benefits of antineoplastons against a wide range of cancers.

Hydrazine Sulfate

Developed in the 1960s by Dr. Joseph Gold, hydrazine sulfate is only now receiving attention for its anticancer effects.

Dr. Gold's discovery of hydrazine sulfate came after years of research into the cancer-wasting syndrome (medically referred to as _cachexia_). Gold knew that most cancer patients do not actually succumb to cancer but to the severe malnutrition and wasting that result from it. So Gold was determined to find out _how_ cancer causes cachexia, and what could be done to stop it.

After conducting numerous experiments, Gold found that cancer cells require large amounts of glucose (or blood sugar) to multiply. He also found that cancer cells only partially burn up the glucose—much like a defective furnace that inefficiently gobbles up fuel oil. And like a faulty stove that creates lots of soot and carbon, cancer cells also create a waste product known as _lactic acid._

In what Gold described as a "sick relationship," lactic acid is changed back into glucose by the liver, where it is again used by cancer cells for fuel. This process robs the body of energy while creating an unlimited supply of glucose for the cancer. The end result is wasting and severe malnutrition.

Eventually Gold discovered hydrazine sulfate as a drug that could block the lactic acid–glucose cycle. He then began using it in cancer treatment with many reports of success.

Gold is the first to admit that hydrazine sulfate is not a "cure" for cancer but an important complement to other therapies. In fact, he believes that most cancer patients should begin a course of hydrazine therapy before major symptoms emerge, such as progressive weight loss.

HYDRAZINE SULFATE UNDER SCRUTINY

Russian scientists conducted one of the largest trials ever on hydrazine sulfate in 1988. Seven hundred forty patients participated in the study; they suffered from a wide range of cancers.

At study's end, many positive effects were noted, including weight gain, better appetite, less pain, increased mobility, and a better quality of life.

Four additional studies conducted at Harborview/UCLA Medical Center in California by Rowan Chlebowski and colleagues supported the Russian findings; again, improvements in weight, appetite, and other parameters of health were observed. But not all studies on hydrazine sulfate have been so positive.

In a recent NCI multi-institutional trial, favorable results were not found, and NCI researchers declared that hydrazine was without therapeutic benefit. However, critics found serious problems with the NCI trials, citing evidence that the test patients were taking additional drugs such as tranquilizers (these are alleged to interfere with the beneficial effects of hydrazine sulfate).

In fact, the U.S. General Accounting Office *did* confirm that tranquilizers, barbiturates, and other drugs were used during the NCI trials, but did not find proof positive that such drugs altered the outcome of the trials.

Recommended Dosage: Consult your physician or qualified health care provider for dosage information. Your physician can also contact the Syracuse Cancer Research Institute, Inc., listed in Appendix 2, for more information on hydrazine sulfate.

Side Effects: When dosage recommendations are followed carefully (including brief rest periods during therapy), adverse side effects are considered very low. In fact, hydrazine sulfate has shown antidepressant and even "euphoric" side effects.

There have been rare instances of nerve damage or nervous system toxicity for some people who have taken hydrazine sulfate incorrectly, or not according to protocol.

Warning: Those taking hydrazine sulfate should be aware of the following precautions: The drug is a

monoamine oxidase (MAO) inhibitor and is incompatible with tranquilizers, barbiturates, alcohol, and other central-nervous-system depressants. (MAO inhibitors are drugs that show antidepressant activity in the brain; among the most common of these drugs are Elavil, Nardil, and Marplan.) Such drugs can destroy the effectiveness of hydrazine sulfate and increase the dangers from adverse side effects.

Foods high in the amino acid tyramine (such as aged cheeses and fermented products) are also incompatible with MAO inhibitors.

Mind-Body Techniques in Cancer Treatment

Many scientists believe that emotions play a critical role in the onset of and prognosis for cancer. The study of emotions and cancer forms the basis of a medical field known as _psychooncology_.

Therapists who are trained in psychooncology use a number of mind-body methods, including _stress reduction_ and _visual imagery_, to help people better cope with and recover from cancer.

DO MIND-BODY METHODS WORK?

Using the mind as a force against cancer is receiving new support from the highly respected science known as _psychoneuroimmunology_ (or PNI). In fact, PNI research is showing that emotional stress can significantly lower immune-system activity, adversely affecting the body's ability to defend against cancer cells. (Stress can also raise the level of prostate-destructive hormones such as _prolactin_.)

Psychologists believe that cancer-fighting immunity can be significantly enhanced via the following mind-body techniques:

STRESS REDUCTION

Because disease recovery can be adversely affected by stress, methods to alleviate stress are considered very important for improving cancer prognosis. In fact, stress can cause a release of hormones in the body that are injurious to prostate tissues.

There are a number of effective techniques that are used to reduce stress. One of the most useful is *progressive relaxation.*

Progressive relaxation is performed by first tensing up, then relaxing the toes and feet; this sequence of tension/relaxation is then repeated with the calves, abdomen, chest, arms, neck, and head until all tension is released from the body. Slow, deep breathing and the visualization of calm, tranquil scenes accompany progressive relaxation.

Patients are asked to practice this technique daily for ten to twenty minutes.

Another method of relaxation that has proved quite helpful is *meditation.* Of the different types used, *transcendental meditation* (or *TM*) is one of the most popular. TM has been clinically shown to slow the heart rate, reduce galvanic skin response (the sweating that occurs during stress), and improve well-being.

To do TM, a key word, phrase, or syllable is repeated over and over until the mind is calmed and tranquillity is achieved throughout the entire body. The word, phrase, or syllable can be meaningless ("mmmmmmm") or something like "one" or "I am one." The important thing is that the utterances be the sole focus of attention.

Progressive relaxation can also be used to help achieve a more tranquil state of TM.

Biofeedback is another stress-reduction technique that has gained in popularity over the years. It involves the monitoring of bodily functions such as heart rate, blood pressure, and brain activity via the use of electrodes and other types of sensors.

With biofeedback, people can literally _observe_ their heart rate and other functions, and then during periods of stress, alter those functions through the use of relaxation techniques. By actually _watching_ one's stress levels go down on a screen or a monitor, a sense of mental and emotional control over the body is established.

There are a number of clinics and health practitioners equipped to offer biofeedback training (see Appendix 2 for a listing).

VISUAL IMAGERY

This technique is used to help patients create mental pictures or symbols that stimulate the body's cancer-fighting forces. Two types of imageries are commonly used, and they're referred to as _aggressive_ and _passive_.

With aggressive imagery, cancer patients envision their body actively and powerfully fighting cancer cells. One example of this technique is found in O. Carl Simonton's best-selling book, _Getting Well Again._ Simonton describes an imagery scheme that consists of an all-empowered immune system and cancer cells that are weak, purposeless, and vulnerable. The powerful, aggressive, and voracious immune system attacks and destroys the cancer cells and then flushes them out of the body.

This type of imagery approach can also be used in concert with cancer treatments. For example, patients undergoing chemotherapy can develop a viewing scheme in which the drugs are poisoning all the vulnerable cancer cells; the healthy cells, on the other hand, are not absorbing the poisons as quickly and are joining in the fight to eradicate cancer from the body.

Some therapists advocate passive imagery—especially

for patients who are uncomfortable with images of aggression or violence. With passive imagery, immune-system cells can be pictured as peaceful and intelligent, their purpose being to disarm and immobilize cancer cells.

Mind-body practitioners emphasize that it's not necessarily the scheme that's important, but how closely one can identify with that scheme—based on one's personal beliefs.

SELF-HYPNOSIS

This form of mental visualization generally involves two steps. First, a state of deep relaxation is attained (as explained under "Stress Reduction"). Second, a set of verbal commands or suggestions is repeated to oneself so that negative thought patterns stored in the subconscious mind can be changed into positive ones. Self-hypnosis can also help cancer patients to overcome or better cope with physical states such as pain.

A few examples of hypnotic suggestions are: "I will not be fearful but will face my prostate cancer with optimism"; "I will not be receptive to pain, because my brain has natural chemicals that can block pain"; "I will not obsess constantly about my disease, but believe in the healing power of my body." Patients are urged to create their own set of suggestions and then to visualize as fully as possible during hypnosis the goals being sought.

PRAYER

Numerous studies are showing prayer to have powerful effects on the body's ability to recover from or better cope with diseases, including cancer.

Two of the most common forms of prayer are *directed* and *nondirected* prayer. Directed prayer entails seeking a specific goal (for example, asking a higher power to remove a tumor from your body). Directed prayer is very similar to visualization in that both use a technique of mentally focusing on a particular goal.

Nondirected prayer involves not asking for anything specific but simply emptying one's thoughts and completely trusting a higher power for healing—whatever that healing may entail.

According to Dr. Larry Dossey, a leading expert in mindbody healing, your choice of prayer should be shaped by your personality. For example, if you are an extrovert, you might prefer more aggressive, goal-oriented imagery and thus choose directed prayer. If you are an introvert, nondirected prayer might suit your temperament better.

How to Choose a Complementary Cancer Clinic

If you are considering treatment at a clinic that specializes in complementary medicine, answering the following questions will help you choose a qualified practitioner:

- _Is the clinic run by a physician?_ If not, who is in charge of administering the treatment, and what are his or her credentials and experience?
- _What are the clinic's remission or cure percentages for prostate cancer?_ This may be a difficult number to identify, because many clinics treat only patients who are in very advanced or incurable stages of cancer. Still, any available survival percentages can serve as a valuable starting point for further evaluation.
- _When a clinic describes "cures" or "remissions," what is it referring to?_ If a cancer patient has been in remission for eight months, this doesn't signify a "cure"—although some less-than-scrupulous clinicians might make such a claim. But a patient who has been in complete remission with no evidence of cancer for three to five years might be said to be cured. (Ac-

cording to the American Cancer Society, some cancers are considered cured after three years and others after five years. Contact the ACS for more specific information.) Another point to consider is whether or not the ''cured'' patient *had cancer in the first place*. For example, there have been instances when people with self-limiting conditions resembling cancer were said to be ''cured'' after the condition reversed itself.

- *Does the clinic offer radiation, surgery, or chemotherapy?* Obviously, complementary cancer clinics emphasize nontoxic treatments that don't generally consist of radiation, chemotherapy, and surgery. However, *the willingness* of an alternative physician or clinician to consider conventional therapies (especially when they are clearly warranted) is an important indicator of credibility.

- *Does the clinic offer medical documentation or published studies to validate the therapy it offers?* If the clinic can't offer you a large body of scientific proof substantiating its therapy, it should be willing to provide you with patient records showing its treatment's possible effectiveness. Ask for copies of these records, if permitted, and show them to your own doctor or other health professional for an independent review. Be very skeptical of any clinic that doesn't wish to share records or answer specific questions about its protocols or treatment results.

CHAPTER TEN

Putting a Complementary Program into Practice

Now that you've read about the many complementary approaches to treating prostate disease, you might very well be wondering exactly *how* to put these approaches into practice. For example, if you have BPH, do you start by taking saw palmetto and zinc? Or do you try a combination of herbs *and* a varied assortment of vitamins, minerals, and amino acids? And let's not leave out homeopathy, special exercises, sex (more or less), and diet modification—truly a wealth of therapies to choose from!

Actually, it's not as complicated as it all sounds. Remember, the natural strategies discussed in this book are *multidisciplinary* and as such are meant to be used together. So it's probably safe to say that pursuing *more* rather than *fewer* complementary treatments would be the better policy.

Your medical history goes a long way in determining the extent and scope of your natural program. For example, if you have very mild BPH and eat a very nutritious low-fat diet, exercise regularly, and are otherwise healthy, you may not need to do a complete lifestyle makeover; perhaps a trial with saw palmetto, zinc, and vitamin B_6 would be enough. On the other hand, if you are overweight, eat a poor diet, and suffer from more pronounced BPH, you will probably need to adopt considerable lifestyle changes—including a highly modified diet, a combination of nutrients and herbs, physical therapies, and other modalities as discussed throughout this book.

If a prostate infection is the main problem, then vitamins, herbs, and other natural treatments that fight infection and bolster immunity would be the obvious strategies to focus on.

Of course, there are no absolutes when planning a complementary program, because everyone's needs are different. In this regard, we can't tell you *exactly* how to go about organizing a treatment plan, but we can share with you a few examples of men with prostate problems who did.

By reading about their medical circumstances, you might gain additional insights into how to better plan and manage your own.

At the end of the chapter, we'll also provide some useful information on how to choose a qualified health practitioner who can help you put a complementary program into practice.

Note: The following case histories are not meant to reflect similarities with your own and should not be used as a basis for self-diagnosis or self-treatment. Always talk to your doctor first before starting any medical program.

So now let's start with Peter's story.

Peter's Story

Peter is a middle-aged advertising executive who leads a fairly active lifestyle; workouts at the spa and afternoon sessions of racquetball are his daily routines. Peter also tries to be conscious about his weight and is the type to regularly monitor his health through yearly medical checkups. But despite Peter's vigilance about exercise and health, he developed problems shortly after his fifty-fourth birthday; frequent nighttime visits to the bathroom and a feeling that he couldn't completely empty his bladder were Peter's main complaints.

At first he rationalized that routine consumption of water right before bedtime was probably the culprit. But after discontinuing this practice, he continued to experience problems. So erring on the side of caution, Peter decided to schedule an appointment with Dr. R., a urologist referred to him by a work associate.

After meeting with Dr. R., Peter was given a series of tests, and they indeed showed something was wrong.

The rectal examination revealed a soft and "mushy" prostate (to use the doctor's word), and Peter's PSA was moderately elevated for a man his age. To lend more accuracy to the PSA, Peter's doctor ordered a transrectal ultrasound and discovered a prostate with a weight range considered normal for Peter's body size. Additional assays of urine and sperm samples showed no evidence of blood or infectious organisms.

Dr. R.'s diagnosis was "mild BPH," and to Peter's relief, there was no evidence of cancer.

Because Dr. R. was a believer in the Hippocratic oath "First, do no harm," he didn't feel that additional tests (such as needle biopsy or cystoscopy) were necessary—at least for the time being. But the doctor did recommend watchful waiting and urged Peter to come back for a complete checkup in three months so that PSA testing and rectal examination could again be performed.

Relieved the problem wasn't serious, Peter decided it would be a good time to start a natural program in the hopes of "normalizing" his prostate before the next checkup.

Peter was aware of the benefits of zinc and saw palmetto and was also interested in other natural approaches for the prostate. But before deciding to embark on such a program, he called Dr. R. for additional feedback.

When asked about natural medicines, Dr. R. was neither "for" nor "against" them. Actually, he didn't feel a natural approach would be harmful, as long as high dosages of potentially toxic substances such as vitamin A and selenium weren't taken. Peter assured him this wouldn't be the case, and so Dr. R. wished him the best—again reminding his patient to return for a checkup in three months.

Peter's next step was to start a therapeutic nutrient regimen, so he purchased a supplement containing 320 milligrams of standardized saw palmetto extract, 25 milligrams of vitamin B_6, 15 milligrams of zinc, and 50 milligrams of African pygeum. (Since Peter wanted 100 milligrams of vitamin B_6 and 90 milligrams of zinc daily, he bought additional supplements of these nutrients to meet his quota.)

Peter also planned to take 2 tablespoons of brewer's yeast daily, for a complete source of amino acids (including alanine, glycine, and glutamine), and fish oil capsules (for a good source of EFAs). Bee pollen was decided against (because of allergies Peter had shown to honey and flower pollen).

Peter was well aware of the role that diet plays in prostate disease, so he kept a journal of his eating habits for one week to determine his fat intake. After writing down his daily food choices and then averaging out the total fat grams eaten, Peter was surprised to learn that 35 percent of his daily calories were coming from fat; apparently he didn't realize that two eggs every morning with "low-fat" sausages, a large salad every afternoon with wedges of cheese (and classic French dressing), and "just one" doughnut after supper could boost his daily fat calories considerably—despite his emphasis on "healthy eating."

Because he didn't feel his "mild BPH" warranted a very low fat diet, Peter decided on a regimen of 25 percent calories from fat. To help him meet his goal, Peter followed the healthy food choices outlined by the USDA food pyramid. He also followed more specific guidelines for prostate disease (as outlined in the diet plan for men with chronic BPH in Chapter 5).

Daily servings of fruits, soy-based foods, vegetables, and fiber, and generous amounts of "detoxifying" foods such as garlic, crucifers, and onions all became integral to Peter's health program. To further optimize his diet, Peter eliminated red meat and dairy products, and focused on healthy alternatives (such as tofu, vegetable casseroles, and moderate portions of lean white meats, including chicken and pork loin).

At the end of the day, Peter went to the local gym and performed a fifteen-minute aerobic workout—using his target heart rate as a guide. He also took advantage of the gym's Jacuzzi and cold baths and used them in rotation to help reduce prostate enlargement and stimulate circulation (see Chapter 6 for information on rotation baths).

Peter carefully followed his multidisciplinary program for several weeks but didn't notice much change. However, by the second month of treatment, things appeared to be changing for the better. For example, Peter's nighttime visits to the bathroom abated considerably, and he no longer had the sensation that his bladder wasn't emptying fully. Equally impressive, his regularly scheduled checkup with Dr. R. showed a reduction in prostate size and a normalizing of the PSA.

Peter continues taking his saw palmetto supplement daily

but has lowered his dosages of vitamin B_6 and zinc. He also watches his diet very carefully and at this time continues to be healthy.

Kevin's Story

Although he was just thirty-six years old, Kevin was not in the best of health. Overweight and sedentary, Kevin worked as a private security consultant and spent most of his time behind a computer or on the telephone; he rarely exercised, and his dietary staples were processed "junk foods," TV dinners, and quick snacks to keep him "going."

For Kevin, colds, allergies, and sinus problems were almost a weekly event, and it wasn't unusual to see several bottles of antihistamine tablets and pills strewn across his desk. On one occasion, his wife—who was a nurse—noticed that Kevin had also been taking an over-the-counter pain medication. When asked why, Kevin explained that he'd been experiencing "pain after urination." There were also days when Kevin felt a "sudden urge" to return to the bathroom, as well as a "sore" feeling in his perineal area.

Kevin's wife suggested he seek medical advice promptly, so an appointment was made with the couple's longtime physician, Dr. M.

Because Kevin was only thirty-six, his doctor wasn't overly fearful of cancer and, based on the history given, suspected a prostate infection. Tests—including rectal examination and PSA—were conducted, and they confirmed the doctor's suspicions: Kevin had chronic prostatitis caused by an infection, with BPH as a secondary condition.

Unlike acute prostatitis, which typically responds well to antibiotics, the chronic form is more difficult to treat. But Dr. M. still felt a course of medication was indicated, so he prescribed the powerful antibiotic _ciprofloxacin_. He also told Kevin to stop taking antihistamine drugs immediately, drink 8 glasses of cranberry juice or water daily, and to call him in one week.

After a week of therapy, Kevin's urinary-tract symptoms subsided somewhat, although the doctor still found evidence of moderate prostate enlargement. Kevin was puzzled, but the doctor explained that with chronic prostatitis, enlargement could remain even though the infection was treated. In addition, infectious symptoms could return, and the best that could be done was to monitor the situation through watchful waiting.

Dr. M. recommended that Kevin go on a healthier diet, do some moderate exercise, and try to keep his overall health strong. He also suggested a hot bath every night for ten to twenty minutes to help open up the urinary passages. Beyond that, nothing else was prescribed, and a return appointment was scheduled for six months.

Kevin's infection now appeared to be under control, but his BPH continued bothering him. Fearful that his condition would worsen and that further treatments—including surgery—might eventually become necessary, Kevin decided to launch what he termed a "preemptive strike." He would begin a comprehensive program of "vitamins, nutrients, and diet" in the hopes that his prostate problems would clear up by the next checkup. (He'd been meaning to go on a diet for a long time anyway, and this would be a perfect opportunity to do so.)

With his wife's help, Kevin planned a diet regimen that consisted of only 20 percent daily calories from fat. (Because he was significantly overweight _and_ suffered from prostate disease, Kevin felt that a diet based on the lower end of the fat-recommendation guidelines given in Chapter 5 would be best.)

Knowing how easily he was tempted by junk foods, Kevin and his wife "overhauled" their refrigerator and pantry, stocking them with appetizing low-fat items, tasty whole-grain breads and cereals, fresh fruit, healthy low-fat snacks, and unsweetened organic fruit and vegetable juices.

Tuna, salmon steak, grouper, and other flavorful fish selections would become Kevin's main supply of nonmeat protein—as well as an excellent source of EFAs.

Kevin's nutrient regimen consisted of 320 milligrams of saw palmetto, 50 milligrams of pure bee propolis extract, 90 milligrams of zinc, and 100 milligrams of vitamin B_6. In addition, supplemental vitamin C powder (taken to bowel tolerance), echinacea capsules (taken according to labeling instructions), and coenzyme Q10 (in a dosage of 50 milligrams daily) were included to help fight infection and strengthen immunity.

Kevin also decided that the addition of homeopathic medicines to his program would be worth a try. (He knew that these medicines wouldn't interfere with the other natural substances he was taking and that different medicines could be tried with no concerns about side effects.) So Kevin matched his symptoms (pain after urination, perineal discomfort with a frequent urge to urinate) with their respective medications (Causticum, Chimaphila). He used a homeopathic medicine chart similar to the one provided in Chapter 4 and decided that 30X potencies would be the best to take.

After diligently following his complementary program for two months, Kevin began noticing gradual improvements. For example, he no longer felt soreness in the perineal area, and the sensation of frequently having to urinate diminished. Finally, he had spent a full week without *any* symptoms and realized that he had almost forgotten what it was like to feel "normal."

Kevin also noticed an improvement in his *overall* health; besides losing some of the weight he had long hoped to, Kevin didn't tire as easily, didn't become breathless after only mild exertion, and seemed to be free of colds and sinus problems.

Kevin's progress was certainly made evident during his next physical; follow-up sperm and urine samples showed no infection, and rectal examination revealed a relatively normal prostate. At this time, Kevin continues in good health—and continues avoiding junk foods like the plague.

Carl's Story

At seventy-five, Carl was considered the envy of his family and friends. A hairstylist for fifty years, Carl hadn't slowed down at all, was vibrant and active, and maintained a steady stream of weekday customers in his corner barbershop.

Weekends were filled with social and recreational activities that included bowling, dancing, and long evening walks. In addition to his regular exercising, Carl believed in healthy eating and moderate drinking. He also saw his doctor every six months for regular PSA and rectal examinations and was a firm believer in prevention's being the best form of medicine.

Carl's vigilance about regular checkups proved well worth it when, after a routine physical, several tiny nodules were found on his prostate. During the examination, Carl's primary physician (whom we'll call Dr. Y.) also found a PSA reading of 12 (6.5 or less is considered normal for a man of seventy-five) and microscopic blood cells in the urine. Suspecting cancer, Dr. Y. ordered a needle biopsy, and the test indeed showed the nodules to be malignant.

According to Dr. Y., Carl's cancer was in an "early

stage,'' and all indications were that the tumors had not extended outside of the prostate. Based on this information, Dr. Y. outlined two medical strategies that he felt were the most appropriate for Carl to consider: one was ''radical surgery'' to completely remove the prostate, and the other, watchful waiting in which the prostate would be left alone and Carl's condition carefully monitored.

Dr. Y. explained that several studies—one of which had recently appeared in *Journal of the American Medical Association*—showed that older men who'd had radical surgery survived only slightly longer than men who didn't undergo such a procedure (and even this slight difference in survival was still being debated). The *JAMA* results were particularly true for men with slow-growing cancers (such as Carl's were found to be).

Dr. Y. went on to explain that both options did have their ''pros and cons.'' For example, prostate surgery could lead to permanent complications, including impotence and chronic urinary problems—obstacles that would significantly impact Carl's active and social lifestyle. But on the other hand, watchful waiting meant the possibility of Carl's tumors' spreading—and *that* would be a very dangerous situation indeed.

Dr. Y. did point out that the ''choice of surgeon'' could greatly improve Carl's odds for a successful operation. He also emphasized that ''careful and regular monitoring'' would lower the risks associated with watchful waiting. (If Carl were to choose watchful waiting, Dr. Y. suggested frequent PSA tests, rectal examinations, transrectal ultrasounds, and biopsies.) Ultimately, Dr. Y. was leaving the decision up to Carl and suggested he take a few days to think about it.

Carl liked and respected Dr. Y. and had always had a good rapport with him. But he felt compelled to be doubly sure of his options before committing to any one and thus scheduled an appointment with a urologist named Dr. B.

After a lengthy examination and a careful review of Carl's medical records, Dr. B. suggested watchful waiting as a "serious option." He based his recommendation on Carl's age, on the grade of tumor (it appeared to be "very slow growing"), and on the fact that surgery could adversely affect Carl's active and busy lifestyle.

Carl was relieved that the two doctors had been in relative agreement, and after several more days of mulling it over, opted for watchful waiting.

Three months after Carl made his decision, an examination showed that his PSA had actually dropped slightly—although the size and characteristics of his tumors hadn't changed. This was certainly acceptable news, but Carl wanted to do more than just sit back and hope for the best; indeed, he felt that by strengthening his body and immune system through natural means, his tumors might recede or at the very least not ever grow any larger. But Carl wasn't quite sure what *type* of natural program he should pursue.

Then one afternoon while leafing through health magazines in his shop, Carl spotted an article about a complementary medical clinic in California. The clinic treated patients with a low-sodium vegetarian diet (based on the Gerson diet), immune-boosting vaccines, intravenous vitamins and minerals, and medications that were considered "less toxic" than standard medicines (similar therapies are discussed in Chapter 9). According to the article, favorable results were being reported by some cancer patients, and this especially caught Carl's attention.

After reading through a prospectus and a brochure, Carl learned that the clinic's staff consisted of two board-certified physicians, a naturopathic doctor, and a registered nurse. In addition, treatments offered at the clinic were used in conjunction with standard therapies, and the clinic's policy was to work with outside physicians when necessary. Carl was further impressed that a staff member had taken the time to speak with him on the telephone and answer all his questions, and had not made exorbitant claims about "cures" or "miracle treatments."

Carl promised to call the clinic back after speaking with his insurance company (the full complementary program in California would cost $5,000).

Initially, Carl had some doubts about reimbursement—even before contacting the insurance people. Earlier he'd recalled reading in his policy that "only surgery, hormone therapies, or radiation" for prostate cancer would be covered. However, the California clinic didn't treat *cancer* per se but *was* licensed and accredited by the California Medical Association to treat *allergies* and other disorders of the *immune system* (cancer was considered one such disorder, according to the clinic's physicians).

Since Carl had suffered from occasional allergies and had also shown a white blood cell abnormality in previous tests, his pursuit of immunologic therapy was considered medically valid and therefore coverable by insurance. He simply needed to offer proof, and the doctors in California did so after reviewing Carl's medical records.

Pleased that the financial details had been worked out, Carl made the trip out to California and spent a week at the clinic as an outpatient (insurance didn't cover outside living expenses, but Carl had managed to save for an eventual vacation and now used the money accordingly). He finally met with the clinic's staff, gave a detailed and comprehensive history, underwent a number of blood and urine tests, and was then asked to return the following day to begin treatment.

Carl's treatment program included a specially designed

diet that excluded salt, most animal foods, coffee, tea, and alcohol. He was also required to take 8 glasses of freshly pressed vegetable and fruit juices daily. The diet restrictions would be loosened up somewhat after six months.

Additional treatments included the immune-boosting vaccines BCG and gamma globulin, intravenous vitamin C, shark cartilage, high-dose selenium (given in a nontoxic lipid form), and coenzyme Q10. Hydrazine sulfate was also prescribed, and when Carl asked why, his doctor explained that it might interfere with tumor growth. In fact, Carl remembered seeing a number of article excerpts on hydrazine sulfate in the clinic's prospectus.

Carl experienced very mild reactions to treatment, but none that were uncomfortable. For example, the BCG vaccine led to a mild skin reaction, and the vitamin C caused hot flashes, but these effects quickly subsided.

The most difficult part for Carl was the diet, but with the support of staff and of fellow patients, he began feeling more positive about it. In fact, after several weeks, Carl found that his diet wasn't so "radical" after all—though he did have to make some adjustments in his social life. For example, his weekly dance was an occasion to indulge in Polish, Hungarian, and other ethnic foods (many of which are very fatty and salty), but for now these foods were out of the question; instead, Carl was more than happy to bring a chef's salad to his dances—notwithstanding the puzzled looks of his friends.

Carl also chose not to join in the after-bowling bar stop he sometimes made with his fellow players; although he might customarily have only one or at most two drinks, he was on total alcohol restriction and was determined to not put himself in a compromising situation.

Perhaps most difficult of all, Carl had to revise his entire way of looking at and preparing meals. This meant shopping at organic markets and health food stores for the bulk of his foods, getting "used to" a low-salt diet for the next six months, and preparing his own juices in a juicer—per the instructions of his California doctors.

And because he was on a daily maintenance dosage of hydrazine sulfate, Carl could not eat cheese or other fermented foods since these might lead to a dangerous drug reaction.

Several months after beginning his treatment program, Carl began noticing some positive effects. For instance, his energy levels improved (though he was already an energetic person), and his allergies cleared up completely. But perhaps the most surprising news came from his next office visit with Dr. Y.

Although there was no evidence that Carl's cancer had gone into active remission, there were indications that the tumors had "softened." In fact, ultrasound did show a slight diminishing in tumor size. Equally significant, Carl's PSA dropped to 7 from its previous 12, and that was considered a good sign. Additional blood tests also showed a normalization in white blood cell levels and a normally functioning immune system.

Dr. Y. was obviously very pleased, but he cautioned that it would take "several years" of monitoring to gauge Carl's true progress *and* to determine just how much of an effect the complementary program was having. Still, Dr. Y. told his patient to "keep on doing what you're doing," and this was one piece of advice Carl didn't need a second opinion on.

How to Determine If a Therapist Is Right for You

As seen in our previous examples, a program of self-treatment with natural medicines is a feasible option—provided you've first been examined by your physician. However, some people feel more comfortable seeking treatment with a physician or other health care practitioner who specializes in complementary medicine; this is especially true in cases involving more serious diseases such as cancer.

If you are seeking professional advice on complementary medicines, how do you go about finding a qualified and competent practitioner? First and foremost, look for someone who is both qualified _and_ responsive to your needs. The ideal practitioner is one with whom you can freely voice your fears, concerns, and health goals. In this regard, you should be able to freely question any treatments or suggestions that you don't understand or aren't comfortable with, and to also offer your own ideas about possible strategies that you feel may be worth considering.

Pay attention to your therapist's goals and expectations regarding your condition. Is he reasonable in his approach toward treatment? Does he promise an instant "cure," or is your condition one that will take "years" to clear up? (There are seldom instant cures, but medical conditions that are benign shouldn't take years to clear up either.)

Be leery of any treatments or suggestions that seem farfetched or unreasonable; since you've already read about important complementary therapies in this book, you should have a good working knowledge of what to look for and what to expect. Trust your instincts, and don't be afraid to challenge your therapist when an idea or suggestion doesn't seem quite right. On the other hand, your therapist may offer a particular treatment that you're simply not familiar with, and if that's the case, ask about the background of the treatment and about any studies that support it.

A few more questions bear mention: Is your therapist willing to communicate and work with other clinicians you may be consulting? (Not willing to do so should raise a red flag and at least deserves an explanation.) And has the issue of reimbursement been clearly outlined? (Some insurance companies may not reimburse for complementary treatments, so you'll need to have a clear understanding of how you will pay, how much you will be expected to pay, and the type of payment schedule your clinician is willing to let you arrange—if that's what your circumstances require.)

One good place to start looking for a complementary therapist is in your local Yellow Pages. Several listings to check under are "herbs," "holistic practitioners," "homeopaths," "naturopathic physicians," and "nutritionists." In some cases you'll find separate listings for medical doctors who also practice complementary forms of medicine.

Use Appendix 2 of this book to direct you to organizations that can refer you to a complementary practitioner. The appendix also has a separate listing of medical doctors, naturopathic physicians, and clinics that offer specific therapies for prostate cancer (these therapies are discussed in detail in Chapter 9).

APPENDIX 1

Recommended Nutrient Guidelines

GENERAL SUPPLEMENTATION PROGRAM FOR MAINTAINING PROSTATE HEALTH

Nutrient	Optimum Daily Recommended Dosage
Vitamin A	10,000–25,000 IU
Beta-carotene	15,000–30,000 IU
Vitamin B_1	10 mg
Vitamin B_2	10 mg
Vitamin B_3	10 mg
Vitamin B_6	**25 mg**
Vitamin B_{12}	10 mcg
Pantothenic acid	50 mg
Folic acid	400 mcg
Biotin	300 mcg
Lecithin (for biotin and inositol content)	2 tbsp. (granulated form)
Vitamin C	500–1,000 mg
Vitamin D	400 IU

Vitamin E	200–400 IU
Calcium	500 mg
Magnesium	150 mg
Iodine	150 mcg
Selenium	150 mcg
Iron	18 mg
Copper	2 mg
Zinc picolinate	**15–30 mg**

SUPPLEMENTATION PROGRAM FOR BPH OR NONBACTERIAL PROSTATITIS

Follow the general supplementation guidelines for maintaining prostate health. Also, **INCREASE** the dosage of or **ADD** the following nutrients:

Nutrient	*Daily Total*[†]
Vitamin B_6	50–100 mg for the first month, 25–50 mg thereafter
Zinc picolinate	90–120 mg for the first month, 60 mg daily until symptoms improve
Fish oil	180 mg EPA/120 mg DHA, 2 capsules three times daily
Amino Acids	
L-glutamic acid	250 mg three times daily
L-glycine	250 mg three times daily
L-alanine	250 mg three times daily
DL-phenylalanine (for natural pain control)	250 mg one to three times daily
Herbs	
Saw palmetto extract	320 mg
African pygeum	50–100 mg

Nettle   250 mg one to three times
                                            daily

Bee propolis   50–250 mg

Homeopathic
See Chapter 4 for a complete overview.

SUPPLEMENTATION PROGRAM FOR PROSTATE INFECTIONS AND RELATED CONDITIONS

Follow the supplementation guidelines for **BPH** or nonbacterial prostatitis. Also, **INCREASE** the dosages of or **ADD** the following nutrients:

Nutrient	*Daily Total*[†]
Vitamins B_1, B_2, B_3	50 mg
Vitamin B_{12}	500–1,000 mcg twice per week for one month, twice per month thereafter
Pantothenic acid	50–150 mg
Vitamin C	1–10 g (to bowel tolerance)[‡]
Selenium	250 mcg for one month, 150 mcg thereafter
Coenzyme Q10	30–50 mg for first month, 15–30 mg thereafter

Herbs
See Chapter 3 for information on herbal tonics that can help prostate-related infections.

[†]The dosages given represent total amounts. Be sure to include all other dosages from other supplements you may be taking when calculating your daily total.

[‡]Bowel tolerance means that vitamin C is taken in gradually increasing dosages until symptoms such as flatulence, diarrhea, etc.,

develop. When bowel tolerance is reached, the dosage should be scaled back until symptoms subside; this is considered the optimal dose of vitamin C that's right for your body.

A good starting dosage of vitamin C would be 500 milligrams (a half gram). This can be increased to 1,000 milligrams (1 gram), then 1,500 milligrams (1.5 grams), etc., every four hours. If symptoms develop, scale back to the previous dosage.

You might find that the type of vitamin C you take can make a difference in bowel-tolerance symptoms. For example, some people do not tolerate *ascorbic acid* well but are able to take the *crystallized* form of vitamin C. Others are better able to take *sodium ascorbate* (the salt form) or *calcium ascorbate* (the calcium-buffered form).

Note: Cancer patients aren't advised to take extra sodium—especially for long periods of time. Also, people who are already receiving enough calcium in their diet should avoid taking calcium ascorbate.

Warning: Do not discontinue vitamin C abruptly; doing so can result in what's commonly referred to as the rebound effect, in which symptoms may worsen. *Always* discontinue vitamin C gradually.

APPENDIX 2

Important Resources

Mainstream Organizations (for prostate disease)

Prostate Cancer Support Network
300 W. Pratt St., Suite 401
Baltimore, MD 21201
(800) 828-7866

PAACT (Patient Advocates for Advanced Cancer Treatments)
P.O. Box 141695
Grand Rapids, MI 49514-1695
(616) 453-1477

Natural Association for Continence
P.O. Box 8310
Spartanburg, SC 29307
(800) BLADDER

American Urologic Association
1120 N. Charles St.
Baltimore, MD 21201
(410) 223-4310

The Prostatitis Foundation
Information Distribution Center
2029 Ireland Grove Rd.
Bloomington, IL 61704
(309) 664-6222

Complementary Organizations

Herbal Medicine
The American Herbalists Guild
P.O. Box 1683
Soquel, CA 95073
(408) 464-2441

Herb Research Foundation
1007 Pearl St., #200 F
Boulder, CO 80302
(800) 748-2617 or (303) 449-2265

Holistic & Naturopathic Medicine
American Holistic Medical Association
4101 Lake Boone Trail, Suite 201
Raleigh, NC 27606
(919) 787-5146

American Association of Naturopathic Physicians
601 Valley St., Ste #105
Seattle, WA 98109
(206) 298-0126

Center for Natural Medicine, Inc.
1330 39th Ave. SE
Portland, OR 97214
(503) 232-1100

American College for Advancement in Medicine
23121 Verdugo Dr., Ste 204
Laguna Hills, CA 92653

Homeopathy
National Center for Homeopathy
801 N. Fairfax St., Suite 306
Alexandria, VA 22314
(703) 548-7790

Hydrotherapy
Uchee Pines Institute
Agatha Thrash, M.D., codirector
30 Uchee Pines Rd., Suite #1
Seale, AL 36875
(334) 855-4764

Massage
American Massage Therapy Association
820 Davis St., Suite 100
Evanston, IL 60201-4444
(312) 761-2682

International Institute of Reflexology
P.O. Box 12642
St. Petersburg, FL 33733-2642

Reflexology Research Project
P.O. Box 35820, Suite D
Albuquerque, NM 87176
(888) 777-9911

Mind-Body
American Association of Biofeedback Clinicians
2424 S. Dempster Avenue
Des Plaines, IL 60016
(312) 827-0440

The Wellness Community
National Office
2190 Colorado Ave.
Santa Monica, CA 90404
(310) 453-2300

Center for Attitudinal Healing
19 Main St.
Tiburon, CA 94920
(415) 435-5022

American Psychological Association
750 First Street NE
Washington, D.C. 20002
(202) 336-5500

Yoga
American Yoga Association
513 S. Orange Ave.
Sarasota, FL 34236
(800) 226-5859

International Association of Yoga Therapists
109 Hillside Ave.
Mill Valley, CA 94941

Physicians, Clinics, and Organizations That Practice or Advocate Complementary Therapies for Cancer/and or Prostate Disease

Atkins Center for Complementary Medicine
152 East 55th St.
New York, NY 10022
(212) 758-2110

Burzynski Research Institute
12000 Richmond Ave.
Houston, TX 77082
(713) 597-0111 or fax (713) 597-1166
  For treatment information on antineoplastons

Center for Metabolic Disorders
P.O. Box 1134
Dania, FL 33004
(305) 929-4814

Central Coast Holistic Medical Services
32 E. Sola St.
Santa Barbara, CA 93101
(805) 569-5594

The Gerson Institute
P.O. Box 430
Bonita, CA 91908
(619) 585-7600
  Provides information on the original Gerson diet therapy for cancer.

Gerson Research Organization
7807 Artesian Rd.
San Diego, CA 92127-2117
(800) 759-2966
  An offshoot of the original Gerson therapy; provides clinic information on the Gerson diet and other natural therapies for cancer.

James R. Privitera, M.D.
105 North Grandview Ave.
Covina, CA 91723
(818) 966-1618

Hoffman Center
40 E. 30th St.
New York, NY 10016
(212) 779-1744

Keith Block, M.D.
899 Sherman Ave., Suite 515
Evanston, IL 60201
(708) 492-3040

The Kushi Institute
Box 7
Becket, MA 01223
(413) 623-2322 or fax (413) 623-8827
  Provides information and counseling on macrobiotics in cancer treatment.

Livingston Clinic for Allergy and Immunology
3232 Duke St.
San Diego, CA 92110
(619) 224-3515

Lost Horizon Health Awareness Center
P.O. Box 620550
Oviedo, FL 32762-0550
(407) 365-6681

Richard P. Huemer, M.D.
3303 44th St. NE
Vancouver, WA
(360) 696-4405

Schachter and Associates
Two Executive Blvd., Suite 202
Suffern, NY 10901
(914) 368-4700

Simone Protective Cancer Center
123 Franklin Corner Rd.
Lawrenceville, NJ 08648
(609) 896-2646

Syracuse Cancer Research Institute, Inc.
Presidential Plaza
600 East Genesee St.
Syracuse, NY 13202
(315) 472-6616
   The headquarters for research and information on hydrazine sulfate.

The Waisbren Clinic
2315 North Lake Dr., Suite 815
Seton Tower
Milwaukee, WI 53211
(414) 272-1929
   Immunologic vaccine program based on the protocols of Burton Waisbren, M.D.

Where to Order Supplies

Chinese Herbs
The Brian Herb Corporation
9250 Jeronim Rd.
Irvine, CA 92718
(800) 333-HERB

International Traditional Medicines
2017 Hawthorne SE
Portland, OR 97214
(800) 544-7504

Nuherbs Company
3820 Penniman Ave.
Oakland, CA 94619
(800) 233-4307

Conventional Herbs
Nature's Way Products, Inc.
10 Mt. Spring Pkwy.
Springville, UT 84663

Herb Pharm
P.O. Box 116-N
Williams, OR 97544
(800) 348-4372

Homeopathic Remedies
Boericke & Tafel, Inc.
1011 Arch St.
Philadelphia, PA 19107
(800) 876-9505

Boiron-Borneman
1204 Amosland Rd.
Norwood, PA 19074
(800) 258-8823

Hydrazine Sulfate

Physicians can contact the following mail-order companies to order hydrazine sulfate direct:

Great Lakes Metabolics
1724 Hiawatha Court NE
Rochester, MN 55904
(507) 288-2348

Rapier USA, Inc.
P.O. Box 11234
Pompano Beach, FL 33061
(954) 941-7577

References

Introduction

American Cancer Society. *Cancer Facts and Figures.* 1993.

Eisenberg, D. M. et al. "Unconventional Medicine in the United States: Prevalence, Costs and Patterns of Use." *New England Journal of Medicine* 328 (1993):246–52.

Chapter One

Fox, Arnold, M.D. *The Healthy Prostate.* New York: John Wiley & Sons, 1996.

Horton, R. "BPH: A Disorder of Androgen Metabolism in the Male." *J Am Ger Soc* 32 (1984):380–5.

Ask-Upmark, E. "Prostatitis and Its Treatment." *Acta Med Scand* 181 (1967):355–7.

Tammela, T. "Benign Prostatic Hyperplasia: Practical Treatment Guidelines." *Drugs Aging* 10 (May 1997):349–66.

Schaffner, C. P. et al. "Effect of Cholesterol-Lowering Agents," *BPH.* New York: Springer-Verlag, 1983:295.

The Merck Manual: 16th Edition. Rahway, N.J.: Merck Research Laboratories, 1992.

Chapter Two

Fahim, M. et al. "Zinc Treatment for the Reduction of Hyperplasia of the Prostate." *Fed Proc* 35 (1976):361.

Leake, A. et al. "The Effects of Zinc on the 5-alpha Reduction of Testosterone in the Hyperplastic Human Prostate Gland." *J Steroid Biochem* 20 (1984):651–5.

———. "Subcellular Distribution of Zinc in Benign and Malignant Human Prostate: Evidence for a Direct Zinc-Androgen Interaction." *Acta Endocrinol (Copenh)* 105 (1984):281–8.

Grant, J. E. et al. "Effect of Zinc on Androgen Metabolism in the Human Hyperplastic Prostate." *Biochem Soc Trans* 3 (1975):540–2.

Judd, A. M. et al. "Zinc Acutely, Selectively and Reversibly Inhibits Pituitary Prolactin Secretion." *Brain Res* 294 (1984):190–2.

"Effects of Zinc, Vitamin B_6 and Picolinic Acid on Zinc Absorption in the Rat." *J Nutr* 111 (1981):68–75.

Hart, J. P. et al. "Vitamin F in the Treatment of Prostatic Hyperplasia," no 1. Milwaukee: Monograph published by the Lee Foundation for Nutritional Research, 1941.

Scott, W. W. "The Lipids of the Prostatic Fluid, Seminal Plasma and Enlarged Prostate Gland of Man." *J Urol* 53 (1945):312–18.

Dumerau, F. "BPH: Amino Acid Therapy for Symptomatic Relief." *Am J Geriatrics* 10 (1962):426–30.

Feinblat, H. M. et al. "Palliative Treatment of BPH: Value of Glycine, Alanine, Glutamic Acid Combination." *J Maine Med Assoc* 49 (1958):99–102.

Chapter Three

Kaptchuk, T. J. *The Web Has No Weaver*. New York: Contemporary Books, 1983.

Weiner, Michael. *Herbs That Heal*. Cambridge, MA: Quantum Books, 1994.

Champlautt, G. et al. "A Double-blind Trial of an Extract of the Plant Serenoa Repens in BPH." *Br J Clinical Pharmacol* 18 (1984):461–2.

Tosca, A. et al. "Treatment of Obstructive Symptomatology Caused by Prostatic Adenoma with an Extract of Serenoa Repens . . . Double Blind vs. Placebo." *Minerva Urol Nefrol* 37 (1985):87–91.

Legromandi, C. et al. "The Importance of African Pygeum in the Treatment of Chronic Prostate Abnormalities." *Gazz Med It* 143 (1984):73.

Guillemein, P. "Clinical Study on V1326 [an African pygeum preparation] for Adenoma of the Prostate." *Med Practic* 386 (1970):75.

Ranno, S. et al. "Efficacy and Tolerability of Treatment for Adenoma of the Prostate with Tadenan 50 [African Pygeum preparation]." *Progresso Medico* 62 (1986):165.

Tyler, V. E. *Herbs of Choice.* New York: Pharmaceutical Products Press, 1994:84–5.

"Treatment of Benign Prostatic Hyperplasia with Prostat." Monograph published by China Medical University Affiliated to the First Hospital, June 1996.

Rugendorff, E. W. "Results of Treatment with Pollen Extract (Cernilton N) in Chronic Prostatitis and Prostatodynia." *British Journal of Urology* 71 (1993):433–38.

Ohkoshi, M. et al. "Clinical Effect of Cernilton in Chronic Prostatitis." *Acta Urol Jpn* 38 (1992):489–94.

Tierra, Michael. *The Way Of Herbs.* New York: Pocket Books, 1990.

Hong, Yen. *How to Treat Yourself with Chinese Herbs.* New Canaan, Conn.: Keats, 1993.

Chapter Four

Reilly, D. et al. "Is Evidence for Homeopathy Reproducible?" *Lancet* 344 (Dec. 10, 1994):1601–6.

Jacobs, J. et al. "Treatment of Acute Childhood Diarrhea with Homeopathic Medicine: A Randomized Clinical Trial in Nicaragua." *Pediatrics* 93 (May 1994):719–25.

LeRoy, D. et al. "Aspirin at Very Ultra Low Doses in Healthy Volunteers: Effects on Bleeding Time . . . and Coagulation." *Haemostasis* 20 (1990):99.

Day, C. "Control of Stillbirths in Pigs Using Homeopathy." *Veterinary Records* 114 (March 3, 1984):216.

Vozianov, A. F. "Homeopathic Treatment of Patients with Adenoma of the Prostate." *British Homeopathy J* 79 (July 1990):148–51.

Rose, B. *The Family Guide to Homeopathy.* Millbrae, CA: Celestial Arts, 1992.

Chapter Five

Barnard, N. *Eat Right, Live Longer.* New York: Crown, 1995.

Schaffner, C. P. et al. "Effect of Cholesterol-lowering Agents." *BPH.* New York: Springer-Verlag, 1983:295.

Araki, H. et al. "High-Risk Group for BPH." *Prostate* 4 (1983):253–64.

Hamalainen, E. H. et al. "Decrease of Serum and Total Free Testosterone During a Low-Fat, High-Fiber Diet." *J Steroid Biochem* 18 (1983):369–70.

Food Guide Pyramid source: U.S. Department of Agriculture, U.S. Department of Health and Human Services.

Duyff, Roberta Larson, ed. *Complete Food and Nutrition Guide.* New York: The American Dietetic Association, Chronimed Pub., 1996.

Ho, P.J., and Baxter, R.C. "Insulin-like Growth Factor-Binding Protein-2 in Patients with Prostate Carcinoma and Benign Prostatic Hyperplasia." *Clin Endocrinol (Oxf)* 46 (March 1997):333–42.

Eades, Mary D. *The Doctor's Complete Guide to Vitamins and Minerals.* New York: Dell Publishing 1994:28–31.

Ask-Upmark, E. "Prostatitis and Its Treatment." *Acta Med Scand,* 181 (1967):355–7.

Flora S. J. S. et al. "Protective Role of Trace Metals in Lead Intoxication." *Toxicology Letters,* 13 (1982):51–6.

Passwater, R. A. et al. *Trace Elements, Hair Analysis, and Nutrition.* New Canaan, Conn.: Keats, 1983.

Pearson, D., and Shaw, S. *Life Extension.* New York: Warner Books, 1982.

Lindsay, A. *The American Cancer Society Cookbook.* New York: William & Morrow, 1988.

Foods That Harm, Foods That Heal. VA: Reader's Digest, 1997.

Mandell, M. *5-Day Allergy Relief System.* New York: Pocket Books, 1980.

Bragg, P. *The Miracle of Fasting.* Santa Barbara, Calif.: Health Science, 1983.

Chapter Six

Guide to Medical Cures and Treatments. New York: The Reader's Digest Association, Inc., 1996.

The Alternative Advisor. Alexandria, Va.: Time-Life, 1997.

Kindersely, D. *Yoga Mind-Body.* New York: DK Publishing, Inc., 1996.

Christensen, Alice. *Beginning Yoga Manual.* American Yoga Association, 1995.

Chaitow, L. *Prostate Trouble.* London: Thorsons, 1988.

Fox, Arnold, M.D. *The Healthy Prostate.* New York: John Wiley & Sons, 1996.

Laing, W. *The 1996 China Reflexology Symposium Report of the China Reflexology Association.*

Carter, M. *Hand Reflexology.* New York: Parker Publishing Inc., 1975.

Inge, D. *The Art of Reflexology.* Rockport, MA: Element Books, 1992.

Chapter Seven

Fox, A. "The Non-Surgical Treatment of Prostatic Disease." *The Healthy Prostate.* New York: John Wiley & Sons, 1996.

Pierce, V. *The People's Common Sense Medical Adviser.* Buffalo, N.Y.: The World's Dispensary Medical Association, 1936.

Morganstein, S., and Abrahams, A. *The Prostate Sourcebook.* Los Angeles: Contemporary Books, 1996.

Chapter Eight

Dollinger, Rosenbaum, Cable. *Everyone's Guide to Cancer Therapy.* Kansas City: Somerville House, 1994.

"Prostate Cancer May Have Roots in Genetic Defect." *Los Angeles Times* (November 22, 1994):A-30.

Barnard, N. *Eat Right, Live Longer.* New York: Crown, 1995.

Fleming, C. et al. "A Decision Analysis of Alternative Treatment Strategies for Clinically Localized Prostate Cancer." *JAMA* 20 (May 1993):2650–658.

Information for Health Care Professionals, Physicians Data Query, the National Cancer Institute: "Prostate Cancer." Statement no. 208/01229, 1997.

Thompson, I. M. "What Is Watchful Waiting? Does It Make Sense in the Patient Under Age 75?" (meeting abstract) Fifth Annual International Conference: Prostate Cancer–Urothelial Cancer–BPH. Orlando, Fla., March 2–4, 1995.

———. "Radical Perineal Prostatectomy" (meeting abstract). Fifth Annual International Conference: Prostate Cancer–Urothelial Cancer–BPH. Orlando, Fla., March 2–4, 1995:10.

Bruchovsky, N. et al. "Intermittent Androgen Blockade Therapy in Prostate Cancer" (meeting abstract). *Cancer Invest* 13 (Suppl. 1, 1995):46.

Schmidt, J. D. et al. "Treatment of Metastatic Prostate Cancer with Emphasis on Prognostic Factors" (meeting abstract). Fifth Annual International Conference: Prostate Cancer–Urothelial Cancer–BPH. Orlando, Fla., March 2–4, 1995:18–9.

Anscher, M. S. et al. "Combined External Beam Irradiation and External Regional Hyperthermia for Locally Advanced Adenocarcinoma of the Prostate." *Int J Radiat Oncol Biol Phys* 37 (March 15, 1997):1059–65.

Hawatmeh, A. S. et al. "Early Clinical Experience with Percutaneous Cryosurgical Ablation of the Prostate." *Mo Med* 92 (November 1995):705–9.

Bales, G. T. et al. "Short-Term Outcomes After Cryosurgical Ablation of the Prostate in Men with Recurrent Prostate Carcinoma Following Radiation Therapy." *Urology* 46 (November 1995):676–80.

Chapter Nine

Lechner, P., and Kroenberger, I. "Experiences with the Use of Dietary Therapy in Surgical Oncology." *Tropical Nutritional Medicine* 2, band 15, April 1990.

Newbold, Vivian. "Remission of Advanced Malignant Disease: A Review of Cases with a Possible Dietary Factor." *Cancer Free,* compiled by the East West Foundation. New York: Japan Publications, 1991:239.

"Summary of a Retrospective Study of Diet and Cancer of the Pancreas." Tulane School of Public Health and Tropical Medicine, Dept. of Nutrition, 1984/1985.

Cameron, E., and Pauling, L. "Supplemental Ascorbate in the Supportive Treatment of Cancer: Prolongation of Survival Times in Terminal Human Cancer." *Proc Natl Acad Sci U S A* 73 (1976):3685–89.

Pauling, L. *Cancer and Vitamin C.* New York: W.W. Norton, 1979.

Reichman, M. et al. "Serum Vitamin A and Subsequent Development of Prostate Cancer." *Ca Research* 50 (1990):2311–15.

Schrauzer, G. G. et al. "Statistical Associations with Dietary Selenium Intakes." *Bioinorganic Chem* 7 (1977):23–34, 35–56.

Satoh, H. et al. "Antitumor activity of . . . germanium compound, GE132." *Gan To Kagaku Ryoho* 6 (1979):79–83.

Langer, R., and Lee, A. "Shark Cartilage Contains Inhibitors of Tumor Angiogenesis." *Science* 221:185–87.

Waisbren, B. A. "Observations on the Combined Systemic Administration of Mixed Bacterial Vaccines, BCG, Transfer Factor and Lymphoblastoid Lymphocytes to Patients with Cancer, 1974–1985." *J Biol Resp Mod* 6 (1987):1–19.

Moss, R. *Cancer Therapy: The Independent Consumer's Guide.* New York: Equinox Press, 1996:160–5.

Hunter, Beatrice T. "Could Licorice Prevent Cancer?" *Consumers' Research Magazine* 77 (October, 1994):8.

Burzynski, S. et al. "Treatment of Hormonally Refractory Cancer of the Prostate with Antineoplaston AS2-1." *Drugs Exp Clin Res* 16 (1990):361.

Gersanovich, M. et al. "Results of Clinical Evaluation of Hydrazine." *Vopr Onkol* 36(6) (1990):721–26.

Chlebowski, R. "Hydrazine Sulfate Influence on Nutritional Status and Survival in Non-Small-Cell Lung Cancer." *J Clin Oncol* 8(1) (January 1990):9–15.

Statement on the National Cancer Institute's critique of hydrazine sulfate, by the Syracuse Cancer Research Institute ©1996 (all rights reserved).

Holland, J. C. "Behavioral and Psychological Risk Factors in Cancer: Human Studies." *Handbook of Psychooncology.* New York: Oxford University Press, 1989.

Simonton, Carl O. *Getting Well Again: A Step-by-Step Guide to Overcoming Cancer for Patients and Their Families.* New York: Bantam Books, 1978.

Adams, Paul. *The New Self-Hypnosis.* Hollywood, Calif.: Wilshire Publishing Co., 1967.

Dossey, Larry. *Healing Words.* San Francisco: Harper, 1993.

Chapter Ten

Fleming, C. et al. "A Decision Analysis of Alternative Treatment Strategies for Clinically Localized Prostate Cancer." *JAMA* 20 (May 1993):2650–58.

Glossary

Alpha blockers: Drugs that are typically prescribed for high blood pressure. Alpha blockers have also been found to relax tissues within the prostate gland, thereby reducing swelling. Usually alpha blockers are prescribed to men who have BPH *and* high blood pressure.

Anal-digital examination: Direct finger examination of the prostate via the rectum.

Androgen suppressors: Drugs that interfere with the production of testosterone.

Antiandrogens: Drugs that are used to prevent testosterone production in the adrenal glands. Antiandrogens are usually combined with drugs known as *LHRH agonists* in the medical management of prostate cancer (see also **LHRH agonists**).

Antioxidant: A nutrient or other chemical substance that prevents the oxidation of fats in the body. Oxidation can lead to the formation of free radicals.

Ascorbic acid: The acid version of vitamin C.

BPH (benign prostatic hyperplasia): Noncancerous abnormal growth of prostate tissues, resulting in enlargement.

Beta-carotene: A nutrient that is chemically related to vitamin A. Beta-carotene performs many of the same functions and is also converted into vitamin A in the body as needed.

Bowel tolerance: The threshold dosage at which a substance such as vitamin C causes bloating, diarrhea, and other bowel-related symptoms.

Cachexia: The progressive weight loss and malnourishment that is seen in diseases such as AIDS and cancer.

Cystitis: Inflammation of the urinary bladder, usually caused by a bacterial infection.

Detoxification: Process whereby the body is "cleansed" of toxins and other harmful substances. Naturopathic physicians use vitamins, minerals, and diet as a means of detoxification.

Dihydrotestosterone (DT): A by-product of the male sex hormone testosterone. DT has been found to bind with prostate cells, leading to an overgrowth of tissues. DT levels begin to increase during the fifth and sixth decades of life (see also **5-alpha reductase**).

Dysuria: Painful or difficult urination.

Edema: A buildup of fluid in bodily tissues.

5-alpha reductase: A key enzyme responsible for converting testosterone into dihydrotestosterone. Zinc has been found to inhibit the effects of 5-alpha reductase.

Flare-up: Usually benign symptoms occurring during the course of a food fast. Flare-ups are considered a sign that the body is becoming detoxified.

Free radical: A dangerous molecule that forms when fats combine with oxygen. Free radicals can damage healthy cells and lead to a number of diseases, including cancer and hardening of the arteries.

Frequency: An abnormal increase in the need or urge to urinate *not* caused by excessive drinking of fluids.

Hematuria: Blood in the urine. Hematuria can be *gross* (the blood is visible with the naked eye) or *microscopic* (detected only via a microscope).

Hytrin: An alpha-blocking drug used to treat prostate enlargement.

Isoflavones: Powerful food chemicals found in beans, peas, and soy products; isoflavones have been found to inhibit the formation of prostate cancer.

Laparoscopic lymphadenectomy: The removal of abdominal lymph nodes via a long slender tube inserted into the abdomen.

Law of Similars: The central premise of homeopathy, which stipulates that a disease symptom can be alleviated by taking an extremely small dosage of medicine that under healthy circumstances (and in larger dosages) would cause the same symptom.

LHRH (luteinizing hormone-releasing hormone) agonists: Drugs that are used to prevent the testicles from making testosterone. LHRH agonists are used in the medical management of prostate cancer and are sometimes combined with *antiandrogens* to completely shut down male sex hormone production (see also **antiandrogens**).

Liposterolic extracts: The primary therapeutic ingredients found in saw palmetto berries. A concentration of 85 to 95 percent liposterolic extract is considered effective for reducing prostate enlargement.

Lycopenes: Powerful chemicals found in tomatoes and, to a lesser extent, in citrus fruits; lycopenes have been found to inhibit the formation of prostate cancer.

Lymph node sampling: Procedure in which surgeons examine abdominal lymph nodes to see if there is any evidence of metastasized prostate cancer. Lymph node sampling is usually performed before or during radical prostate surgery.

Monoamine oxidase (MAO) inhibitors: A class of drugs used in the treatment of depression. (The cancer drug hydrazine sulfate has been classified as an MAO-type drug). MAOs can be very dangerous when taken with beer, wine, cheese, other fermented products, or other products containing the amino acid tyramine.

Mother tincture: In homeopathy, the original mixture of a particular medicine. The mother tincture is considered to be the weakest and smallest of all homeopathic dosages.

Nocturia: Frequent urination occurring during the night.

Nonbacterial prostatitis: Inflammation of the prostate not caused by a known infectious agent such as *Klebsiella* or *Escherichia coli.*

Orchiectomy: Removal of the testicles. This procedure is used to stop testosterone production—an important factor in the growth of prostate cancer. Orchiectomies are performed far less often today than they once were.

Oxalates: Substances found in urine that are linked to the formation of kidney stones. Some patients with kidney disease are advised against eating oxalate-rich foods.

Perineal heaviness: A feeling of discomfort in the perineal region (the area between the scrotum and the anus) sometimes caused by an enlarged prostate.

Picolinic acid: A key substance necessary to break down zinc in the intestinal tract. As men age, picolinic acid levels become lower, and the ability to absorb zinc diminishes.

Placebo: An inactive, harmless substance that is prescribed as if it were a real medicine. Placebos are sometimes used in controlled studies as a means of evaluating real versus imagined responses to the actual medicine being tested.

Potentized: In homeopathy, the process of diluting a medicine with alcohol or water so that its therapeutic strength is increased.

Prolactin: A pituitary hormone that is injurious to prostate tissues. Prolactin levels can sometimes become elevated during periods of emotional or psychological stress.

Propolis: The primary ingredient in bee pollen; it shows the most therapeutic activity against benign prostate disease.

Proscar: Androgen-suppressing drug used in the treatment of prostate enlargement.

Prostaglandins: Natural substances in the body that act as chemical messengers. Prostaglandins can reduce inflammation in the prostate but under certain unhealthy conditions cause inflammation.

Prostat: Synthetic drug made from bee pollen and used in the treatment of BPH.

Prostate volume: The size of the prostate as determined by ultrasound. Prostate volume is a useful measurement for helping to determine the accuracy of tests such as the PSA.

Prostatic capsule: The prostate and its underlying areas. Tumors that extend outside of the prostatic capsule are considered less localized and thus not as curable as tumors occurring inside of the capsule.

Prostatic urethra: The small tube inside the prostate through which urine and sperm are carried.

Prostatitis: Inflammation of the prostate, usually caused by a bacterial infection. Symptoms can be similar to those of BPH (in the *chronic* form of prostatitis) but can also be more severe (in the *acute* form).

PSA test: A commonly used test that evaluates levels of a protein known as *prostate-specific antigen;* when PSA levels are elevated, it is a possible indication—but not proof—of prostate cancer. The PSA is not an entirely accurate test, because variations in prostate size can lead to erroneous readings.

PNI (psychoneuroimmunology): The study of how emotions and personality influence the onset of or susceptibility to diseases such as cancer.

Psychooncology: The science that examines ways of coping with and treating cancer via psychological and spiritual methods.

RPP (radical perineal prostatectomy): Removal of the prostate through an incision in the perineum (the area located between the scrotum and the anus).

RRP (radical retropubic prostatectomy): Removal of the prostate through an incision made in the abdomen.

Rebound effect: An adverse reaction that sometimes occurs when a nutrient or other substance is suddenly discontinued after a period of use. Vitamin C and coenzyme Q10 are two nutrients that can result in the rebound effect after sudden discontinuance.

Reflex zone: In reflexology, specific areas of the body (especially the hands and feet) that are said to act as energy pathways. When these pathways become "blocked," energy flow is disrupted, leading to a state of "disharmony" and possibly illness.

Resectoscope: A tube that is used to remove enlarged prostate tissues (see also **TURP**). The resectoscope consists of an outer and inner tube; the outer tube remains stationary inside the urethra while the inner tube is moved back and forth to scrape off the selected tissues.

Residual urine: Urine that remains in the bladder after voiding. Residual urine is often a symptom of prostate disease.

Retrograde ejaculation: The passage of sperm through the bladder and out into the urine. Certain procedures such as TURP can lead to retrograde ejaculation.

Rotation bath: Alternating use of hot and cold baths. Rotation baths are sometimes recommended for men with BPH or for those recovering from prostatitis.

Seminal fluid: A thick whitish secretion that contains sperm and also secretions from the prostate gland. Seminal fluid nourishes sperm and helps transport it out of the body during ejaculation.

Sodium ascorbate: The salt version of vitamin C.

Sterols: Unsaturated alcohol-like chemicals found in African pygeum and other plants. Sterols have shown therapeutic effects against urologic diseases such as BPH.

Testosterone: The male sex hormone. Testosterone has been implicated in the abnormal growth of prostate tissues (see also **dihydrotestosterone**).

TUBD (transurethral balloon dilatation): A method used to open up constricted urinary passages via the expansion of a balloonlike device.

TUIP (transurethral incision of the prostate): A technique involving surgical separation of the urethra from the enlarged tissues surrounding it. A *resectoscope* is used to perform the TUIP.

TULIP (transurethral laser-induced prostatectomy): Reduction of swollen prostate tissues using laser-generated energy.

TUMT (transurethral microwave thermotherapy): A technique that delivers bursts of heat energy into swollen prostate tissues through a water-cooled catheter.

TUNA (transurethral needle ablation of the prostate): A procedure that uses ultrasound to reduce prostatic swelling; the ultrasound is discharged through special needles inserted into the prostate.

TURP (transurethral resection of the prostate): One of the most common procedures used to treat BPH. The TURP is performed by inserting a special tube through the penis and into the prostate; pieces of enlarged prostate tissues are then located and removed (see also **resectoscope**).

Urethritis: Inflammation of the urethra, the tube that carries urine from the bladder and out through the penis. Bladder and kidney infections are common causes of urethritis.

Urinary frequency: A greater-than-normal urge to void—*without* an increase in normal daily urinary output. Urinary frequency is often a sign of prostate disease as well as infections of the bladder or the urethra.

Urinary incontinence: An inability to hold back urine. A number of factors can cause incontinence, including bladder damage resulting from severe BPH and prostate surgery.

Vas deferens: The tube that carries sperm from the testes to the top of the bladder and down into the prostate.

VLAP (visual laser ablation of the prostate): Similar to the TULIP, VLAP uses a visually guided probe to discharge laser energy on enlarged prostate tissues.

Watchful waiting: A medical protocol in which a patient is not treated for a disease but is observed to see if the disease progresses. In cases of prostate cancer that grow very slowly (as often seen in older men), watchful waiting is sometimes considered the best strategy.

Zinc picolinate: A form of zinc that shows therapeutic effects against BPH (see also **picolinic acid**).

Index

Abstinence, sexual, 91–93
Achyranthes bidentata, 45
Aconitum, 45
Acupuncture, 43
Acute prostatitis, 9
Aerobics, 76–78
African pygeum, 31–34, 39
Aggressive visual imagery, 129
Agriculture, U.S. Department of, 61
AIDS (acquired immune deficiency syndrome), 16
Alanine, 20–22
Alcohol, 4, 17, 65, 67, 70, 72, 78
Alisma plantago, 45
Aloe, 52
Aloe emodin, 119
Alpha blockers, 8
American Cancer Society, 132
American Dietetic Association, 60, 63
American Urologic Association, 154

Amino acids, 11, 20–23, 36
Anal-digital examination, 5, 96, 97
Anal intercourse, 9
Androgen suppressors, 8
Anecdotal evidence, 13, 42
Anesthesia, 6
Annual physical examination, 5
Antiandrogens, 103–104
Antibiotics, 9–10, 17
Antihistamines, 4, 67
Antineoplastons, 123–124
Antioxidants, 23–24, 35, 58
Apis mellifica, 52
Ascorbic acid, 24
Aspirin, 20, 50
Astragalus, 27, 42
Austrian Department of General Surgery, 109

Back pain, 9, 53
Bactrim, 9
Baryta carb, 52
Baths, 87–88

BCG, 118
Bee pollen, 36–39
Beer, 65
Benign prostatic hyperplasia
    (BPH), 4
    aerobics and, 76–78
    diet and (*see* Diet)
    herbal medicine for (*see*
        Herbal medicine)
    homeopathy and, 50–54
    hydrotherapy and, 87–88
    kegels and, 82–83
    reflexology and, 83–87
    sexual activity and, 89–93
    standard treatments for, 5–7
    supplements for (*see*
        Supplements)
    symptoms of, 5
    yoga and, 79–82
Benzoapyrenes, 65
Beta-carotene, 23, 116
Bicalutamide, 104
Biofeedback, 128–129
Biopsy, 97
Bladder, 3
    infections, 5, 9
Blood tests, 97
Blurred vision, 8
Bone-marrow suppression, 16
Bowel tolerance, 24
BPH (*see* Benign prostatic
    hyperplasia)
Bread, 62, 64
British Homeopathy Journal,
    50
British Journal of Urology, 37
Buchu, 69
Buckthorn, 119
Burdock, 119–120
Burning sensation, 5, 53, 54

Burzynski, Stanislaw, 108,
    123–124

Cachexia, 124–125
Calcium, 13, 25, 35, 36, 65
Calories, 58–60, 66
Cameron, Ewan, 115
Cancer (*see* Prostate cancer)
Cancer-wasting syndrome,
    124–125
Canola oil, 57
Capsules, 28–29
Carotenes, 36, 65
Causticum, 53
Cayenne, 40
Celery seed, 69
Cereal, 62, 64
Chaitow, Leon, 71
Cheese, 62, 63
Chemical addictions, 73
Chemotherapy, 16
Chimaphila, 53
Chinese herbal medicine, 41–
    45
Chinese yam, 27, 45
Chlebowski, Rowan, 126
Chlorophyll, 35, 65
Cholesterol, 4, 32, 61
Chronic prostatitis, 9
Cigarettes, 72, 73, 78
Cinnamon, 45
Cinnamon bark, 43
Cinnamon twig, 27
Cobra posture, 79–80
Coenzyme Q10, 116
Coffee, 67, 70
Cold baths, 87
Complementary approaches,
    107–148
    antineoplastons, 123–124

Complementary approaches
   (*cont.*)
   choice of approach, 131–132
   choice of therapist, 146–148
   dietary interventions, 109–114
   examples of, 134–146
   herbal medicine, 119–123
   hydrazine sulfate, 124–126
   immmunity-boosting cancer
      programs, 117–119
   mind-body techniques, 127–131
   resources, 157–159
   safety of, 108
   supplements, 114–117
Conium, 53
Cork tree bark, 43
Corn oil, 58
Corn silk, 69
Cranberry juice, 69
Cryosurgery, 105–106
Cystitis, 9, 53, 69*n*

Dairy products, 57, 62, 63
Decoctions, 27–28
Detoxification, 65, 75
Diagnostic tests, 5, 8, 31, 96–98
Diet, 55–75
   in cancer treatment, 109–114
   fasting, 56, 67, 70–75
   fat in, 4, 10, 55, 57–64
   Food Guide Pyramid, 61–64
   general guidelines, 56–66
   reading food labels, 60–61
   restaurant food, 65–66
   sample, 67–68, 112–113
Digitalis, 53
Dihydrotestosterone (*see* DT)
Directed prayer, 130–131
Diuretics, 17, 35
   herbal, 69
Diverticulitis, 69
Dizziness, 8
Dogwood tree, 43, 45
Dosages:
   of African pygeum, 33–34
   of amino acids, 22
   of bee pollen, 38
   of buckthorn, 119
   of burdock, 119–120
   of B vitamins, 17–18
   of coenzyme Q10, 116
   of echinacea, 120
   of essential fatty acids
      (EFAs), 19
   of homeopathic medicines,
      46–47, 51–52
   of hydrazine sulfate, 126
   of licorice root, 120
   of nettle, 35–36
   of pau d'arco, 121
   of pokeweed, 121
   of red clover, 122
   of saw palmetto, 29–31
   of selenium, 24
   of shark cartilage, 117
   of vitamin A, 23, 116
   of vitamin C, 24, 115
   of vitamin E (alpha-
      tocopherol), 24
   of zinc, 15
Dossey, Larry, 131
DT (dihydrotestosterone), 14,
   30
Dysuria, 5, 33, 53, 96

Echinacea, 40, 69, 120
Edema, 32
Eggs, 62, 63
Ejaculation, 90
    painful, 5, 9
    retrograde, 6, 7
Ejaculatory failure, 93
Elavil, 127
Electromagnetic properties, 49
E-Mycin, 9
Endorphins, 21
Ephedra, 42
Erection, 3, 101
    problems achieving, 5
Escherichia coli bacteria, 9
Essential fatty acids (EFAs),
    18–20, 36, 64, 67, 70
Essiac tea, 122–123
Estrogen, 103
Eucamia bark, 43
External beam radiation, 102–
    103
Extracts, 28

Fainting spells, 8
Fasting, 56, 67, 70–75
Fat, in diet, 4, 10, 55, 57–64,
    96
FDA (Food and Drug
    Administration), 30, 124
Fiber, 67
Fish, 62, 63
Fish oil, 11, 18, 19
5-alpha reductase, 14
Flare-ups, 74
Flaxseed oil, 19
Flutamide, 104
Folic acid, 13, 16
Food addictions, 73, 75
Food additives, 4, 55

Food and Drug Administration
    (*see* FDA)
Food Guide Pyramid, 61–64
Food labels, 60–61
Food sources:
    of amino acids, 21
    of B vitamins, 17
    of essential fatty acids
        (EFAs), 19
    of zinc, 15
Free radicals, 23, 24, 57, 58,
    66
Fructose, 64
Fruits, 62, 64

General anesthesia, 6
Genetic factors, 96
Germanium, 25, 117
Germanium oxide, 117
Gerson, Max, 110
Gerson Therapy Daily Menu,
    112–113
Getting Well Again
    (Simonton), 129
Gingerroot, 41
Ginkgo, 42
Ginseng, 42
Glucose, 125
Glutamic acid, 20–22
Glycine, 20–22
Gold, Joseph, 124–125
Goldenlocks tea, 43
Goldenseal root, 40
Goserelin, 104
Grams (g), 12
Gravelroot, 39, 40

Hahnemann, Samuel, 47
*Handbook of Chinese Healing
    Herbs, A* (Reid), 45

Hematuria, 96
Herbal medicine, 26–45
  African pygeum, 31–34, 39
  bee pollen, 36–39
  buckthorn, 119
  burdock, 119–120
  in cancer treatment, 119–
    123
  capsules, 28–29
  Chinese, 41–45
  combinations, 39
  decoctions, 27–28
  echinacea, 40, 69, 120
  Essiac tea, 122–123
  extracts, 28
  infusions, 28
  licorice root, 40, 120
  nettle, 34–36, 39
  pau d'arco, 120–121
  pokeweed, 119, 121–122
  red clover, 122, 123
  resources, 154, 160
  saw palmetto, 29–31, 39
  tinctures, 28
  tonics, 39–41
Herbal teas, 69
Hero posture, 80
High blood pressure, 8, 78
Homeopathy, 46–54
  dosage, 46–47
  resources, 155, 160–161
Hormone therapies, 8, 10,
    103–104
Hot baths, 87
Hunger-control problems, 73
Hydrazine sulfate, 108, 124–
    126, 161
Hydrogenated oils, 57, 64
Hydrotherapy, 87–88, 155

Hyperthermia, 105
Hytrin, 8

Immune system, 15, 16, 23,
    24
Immunity-boosting cancer
    programs, 108, 117–119
Impotence, 6–8, 54, 93, 101,
    106
Incontinence, urinary, 53, 83
Inflammation (*see* Prostatitis)
Infusions, 28
Insect matter, 48
Insomnia, 23
Intercourse, prolonged, 92–93
International units (IU), 12,
    13
Interstitial radiation, 102, 103
Iron, 35, 120

Juniper berries, 39, 40, 69

Kali bichromicum, 53
Kegel exercises, 82–83
Klebsiella bacteria, 9

Lactic acid, 125
Lapachol, 121
Laparoscopic
    lymphadenectomy (*see*
    LL)
Lard, 64
Law of Similars, 47, 50
Lee Foundation for Nutritional
    Research, Milwaukee, 18
LHRH (luteinizing hormone-
    releasing hormone)
    agonists, 103–104
Liang, Wang, 84
Licorice, 40

Licorice root, 120
Linear alcohols, 32
Linoleic acid, 19
Linseed oil, 19
Lipids, 116
Liposterolic extracts, 30, 31
Liquid nitrogen, 106
Livingstone Clinic Daily
    Menu, 112
LL (laparoscopic
    lymphadenectomy), 101
Lobelia, 41
Luprolide, 104
Lycopodium, 53
Lymph nodes, 101
Lymphoblastoid lymphocytes,
    118

Macrobiotics, 110
    Daily Menu, 114
Magnesium, 13, 25, 35, 65
Magnetic resonance imaging
    (*see* MRI)
Magnolia bark, 27
Mandell, Marshall, 71, 74
Marigolds, 48
Marplan, 127
Marshmallow root, 40
Massage:
    reflexology, 83–87
    resources, 155–156
Masturbation, 90, 93
Meat, 57–58, 62, 63
Medical history, 51
Medications, 8–10, 103–104
Meditation, 128
Medorrhinum, 53
Micrograms (mcg), 12–13
Milk, 62, 63
Milligrams (mg), 12, 13

Mind-body techniques, 127
    biofeedback, 128–129
    meditation, 128
    prayer, 130–131
    progressive relaxation, 128
    resources, 156
    self-hypnosis, 130
    visual imagery, 129–130
Minerals (*see* Supplements)
Mixed bacterial vaccine, 118
Monoamine oxidase (MAO)
    inhibitors, 127
Monounsaturated fats, 57, 58
Mother tincture, 48
MRI (magnetic resonance
    imaging), 98

Narpril, 127
National Association for
    Continence, 153
National Cancer Institute
    (NCI), 105, 124
Nausea, 8
Nettle, 34–36, 39
Nocturia, 5, 21, 33, 53, 99
Nonbacterial prostatitis, 10
Nondirected prayer, 130, 131
Nonestrogen drugs, 103–104
Nonoxalate foods, 70
Nutrient deficiences (*see* Diet)
Nuts, 62, 63

Olive oil, 57
Omega-3 fatty acids (*see*
    Essential fatty acids
    (EFAs))
Orchiectomy, 103
Organic foods, 65n, 67
Orgasm, delayed, 92–93

Over-the-counter medications, 4, 67
Oxalates, 70

PAACT (Patient Advocates for Advanced Cancer Treatments), 153
Palm oil, 64
Palpitations, 8
Parsley root, 40, 41
Passive visual imagery, 129–130
Pasta, 62, 64
Pattern recognition, 49
Pau d'arco, 120–121
Pauling, Linus, 115
Pentacyclic triterpenoids, 32
Perineal heaviness, 33
Perineum, 9, 100, 105
Pesticides, 4, 65*n*, 67, 96
Phenylalanine, 20–23
Phenylketonuria, 22
Phytosterols, 32
Picolinic acid, 15, 17
Pituitary gland, 14
Plantain, 43, 45
Plant sterols, 36
Plow posture, 81
PNI (psychoneuro-immunology), 127
Poison ivy, 48
Pokeweed, 119, 121–122
Polyunsaturated fats, 58, 66
Potassium, 35, 36, 48
Potassium dichromate, 47
Potentized, 48
Poultry, 62, 63
Prayer, 130–131
Progressive relaxation, 128
Prolactin, 14, 20, 127

Propolis, 38
Proscar, 8, 97
Prostaglandins, 18, 32, 64
Prostat, 37
Prostate:
    illustration of, 2
    understanding, 3
Prostate cancer, 95–106
    causes of, 10, 96
    complementary approaches (*see* Complementary approaches)
    cryosurgery and, 105–106
    diagnosis of, 96–98
    hormone therapies and, 103–104
    hyperthermia and, 105
    incidence of, 95
    radiation therapy and, 102–103, 105
    resources, 153–154
    stages of, 99–100
    surgical treatment for, 98–102
    survival rates, 99–100
    symptoms of, 96
    treatment of, 10
    undetected, 95
Prostate Cancer Support Network, 154
Prostate disease (*see* Benign prostatic hyperplasia (BPH); Prostatitis)
Prostate enlargement (*see* Benign prostatic hyperplasia)
Prostate-specific antigen test (*see* PSA)
Prostate volume, 97
Prostatic urethra, 3

Prostatitis:
 chronic and acute, 9
 standard treatments for, 9–10
 symptoms of, 9
Prostatitis Foundation, The, 154
Protein-sparing mechanism, 71, 72
PSA (prostate-specific antigen) test, 5, 31, 96–97
 false readings, 8
Psychoneuroimmunology (see PNI)
Psychooncology, 127
Pulsatilla, 53
Pygeum (see African pygeum)

Radiation therapy, 10, 102–103, 105
Radical perineal prostatectomy (see RPP)
Radical retropubic prostatectomy (see RRP)
Rebound effect, 75, 117
Rectal examination, 5, 96, 97
Red clover, 122
Red Clover Combination, 123
Reflexology, 83–87
Rehmannia, 27, 44, 45
Rehmannia Eight Formula, 44
Reid, Daniel, 45
Resectoscope, 6
Residual urination, 5, 33
Resources, 153–161
Restaurant food, 65–66
Retrograde ejaculation, 6, 7
Rice, 62, 64
Rotation baths, 87–88

Royal jelly, 38
RPP (radical perineal prostatectomy), 100–101
RRP (radical retropubic prostatectomy), 100–101

Sabal serrulata, 53
Safflower oil, 58
Saturated fats, 10, 57–58, 64
Saw palmetto (Serenoa repens), 29–31, 39, 97
Saw Palmetto Formula, 39
Selenium, 13, 24, 116
Self-hypnosis, 130
Semen, 3, 90–92
Semifast, 72, 73
Seminal fluid, 3
Sexual activity, 3, 89–93
Shark cartilage, 117
Side effects:
 of African pygeum, 33–34
 of amino acids, 22–23
 of bee pollen, 38–39
 of buckthorn, 119
 of burdock, 120
 of coenzyme Q10, 117
 of cryosurgery, 106
 of essential fatty acids (EFAs), 20
 of hormone therapies, 8, 103, 104
 of hydrazine sulfate, 126
 of licorice root, 120
 of nettle, 36
 of pau d'arco, 121
 of pokeweed, 122
 of radiation therapy, 102–103
 of red clover, 122
 of saw palmetto, 29–31

Side effects (*cont.*)
  of standard treatments for
    BPH, 6, 7
  of surgical procedures, 100,
    101
  of vitamin A, 23, 116
  of vitamin C, 24, 115
  of vitamin E (alpha-
    tocopherol), 24
  of zinc, 16
Simonton, O. Carl, 129
16 Herb Combination, 44–45
Snake venom, 48
Sodium selenite, 24
Soy-based foods, 65, 67
Soybean oil, 58
Spinal anesthesia, 6
Staphysagria, 54
Starvation, 72
Sterols, 33–34
Stinging nettle (*see* Nettle)
Stress reduction, 127–129
Sudafed, 42
Sugar, 64, 72
Sulfur, 48, 65
Sunflower oil, 58
Supplements:
  amino acids, 11, 20–23
  buying and using, 25
  B vitamins, 11, 13, 16–18
  calcium, 13, 25
  dose equivalents, 12–13
  essential fatty acids (EFAs),
    18–20
  germanium, 25
  magnesium, 13, 25
  recommended guidelines,
    149–152
  vitamin A, 13, 23, 116

  vitamin C, 13, 23–24, 35,
    36, 69, 75, 114–116
  vitamin E, 13, 24
  zinc, 11–17, 64, 67, 70
Surgical treatment, 98–102
Sweets, 62, 63
Swimming, 77
Synthetic penicillins, 9

Target heart rate, 77–78
T-cell function, 120
Tea, 67, 70
Testicles, 3
  surgical removal of, 103
Testosterone, 4, 8, 10, 14, 96,
    104
Thuja occidentalis, 54
Tierra, Michael, 40
Tinctures, 28
Tomatoes, 65
Tonics, herbal, 39–41
Total fast, 72, 73
Toxic chemicals, 4, 23, 55
Tranquilizers, 126
Transcendental meditation
    (TM), 128
Transfer factor, 118
Tree peony, 45
TUBD (transurethral balloon
    dilation), 7
Tuckahoe, 45
TUIP (transurethral incision of
    the prostate), 7
Tulane School of Public
    Health, 110
TULIP (transurethral laser-
    induced prostatectomy), 8
TUMT (transurethral
    microwave
    thermotherapy), 8

TUNA (transurethral needle ablation of the prostate), 7
Turbinado sugar, 64
TURP (transurethral resection of the prostate), 6–7
Tyramine, 127

Ultrasound, 7, 97, 98
Urethra, 3
Urethritis, 9, 69*n*
Urinalysis, 96
Urinary incontinence, 53, 83
Urinary tract infections, 5, 9, 53
Urination, 3
  blood in urine, 96
  burning sensation, 5, 53, 54
  delayed, 21
  difficulty in starting, 5, 53, 96
  dribbling, 33, 35, 52, 53
  frequency, 5, 9, 21, 33, 53, 54, 96
  incomplete emptying, 5, 9, 96
  nighttime, 5, 21, 33, 53, 96
Uva-ursi, 39, 40, 69

Vaccines, 117–119
Vas deferens, 3
Vegetable oil, 58
Vegetables, 62–64
Visual imagery, 82, 127, 129–130

Vitamin A, 13, 35, 116
Vitamin B, 11, 13, 16–18
Vitamin C, 13, 23–24, 35, 36, 69, 75, 114–116
Vitamin D, 13
Vitamin E (alpha-tocopherol), 13, 24
VLAP (visual laser ablation of the prostate), 8

Waisbren, Burton, 118
Walking, 77
Walnut, 43
Walsh, Patrick, 102
Warm baths, 87
Watchful waiting, 10, 98
Water, drinking, 67
Way of Herbs, The (Tierra), 40
Weight, 58
White blood cell count, 16
Whole body hyperthermia, 105
Wild hops, 48
Wound healing, 15

Yin and yang, 41, 42
Yoga, 79–82, 156
Yogurt, 62, 63

Zinc, 11–17, 64, 67, 70
Zinc citrate, 16
Zinc picolinate, 16

About the Author

Ron Falcone is a freelance journalist who writes about health, nutrition, and cancer treatment.

His first book, *The Complete Guide to Alternative Cancer Therapies* (New York: Carol Publishing Group, 1994), is considered one of the more balanced and authoritative works on alternative cancer therapies. *Natural Medicine for Prostate Problems* is Mr. Falcone's third book.

Mr. Falcone's articles have appeared in numerous natural-health magazines.

The writer lives in Sanford, Florida, with his wife and their three children.